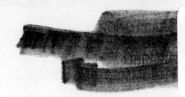

What Doctors Say About This Book

"A revolutionary book that reviews the latest information about, and therapies for, male impotence. A must for doctors, therapists, and patients."

— Mitchell L. Gaynor, M.D.
  Associate Director of Strang-Cornell Cancer Prevention Center and author of *Healing Essence*

"This well researched and clearly written book should add immeasurably to the public's understanding of the once taboo subject of impotence. The medical information presented is factual and well organized. . . . Helps greatly in establishing a meaningful dialogue between patient and doctor."

— Edward C. Muecke, M.D.
  Clinical Professor of Urology, Cornell University Medical School

"A welcome antidote to the accumulated ignorance of a subject vital to the mutual understanding of both sexes, this book should be reassuring to men and to the women who love them. It answers questions traditionally unaddressed by physicians and unasked by their uneasy patients."

— Ruth J. Jacobowitz
  Author of *150 Most-Asked Questions About Midlife Sex, Love and Intimacy* and columnist for *Your Health* magazine

"Factual, yet easily read, this book deals with questions you wouldn't or couldn't ask. Well worth a weekend of reading."

— John Coleman, M.D.
  Associate Professor of Urology, Cornell University Medical School

RECLAIMING
MALE
SEXUALITY

RECLAIMING
MALE
SEXUALITY

A Guide to Potency, Vitality, and Prowess

GEORGE RYAN

Foreword by Arnold Melman, M.D.

M. EVANS AND COMPANY, INC.
New York

M. Evans and Company, Inc.
216 East 49th Street
New York, New York 10017

Library of Congress Cataloging-in-Publication Data

Ryan, George
    Reclaiming Male Sexuality : a guide to potency, vitality, and
prowess / George Ryan
        p.   cm.
    Includes bibliographical references and index.
    ISBN 0-87131-809-1 (pbk.)
    1. Impotence—Popular works.   I. Title
RC889.R93   1997
616.6'92—dc20   96-34928
                                                          CIP

Design and composition by *John Reinhardt Book Design*

WARNING—DISCLAIMER

Contents

Contents

PART III

WHAT YOU CAN DO WITH PROFESSIONAL HELP

Foreword

Male sexual dysfunctions is a problem that affects twenty to thirty million men in the United States. Shifts in political correctness of discussing not only sex, but problems with the act of sex, have allowed public discussion of the subject on radio, television, and the written media.

Despite the recent openness of discussion in the media, however, the dilemma remains for the man with the problem. With whom can he discuss his disability, his loss of his maleness, his machismo? Wives, friends, internists, or family physicians are not often consulted by sexually dysfunctional men. So the problem becomes one of finding a trusted professional who can administer the necessary guidance and help. It has been estimated that only 5 to 10 percent of men with sexual dysfunction actually seek medical help for the problem. Many become easy prey to prolifically advertised nostrums and false aids that have accompanied the rise in media attention.

Clearly, the greater his knowledge, the greater the chance the man with sexual dysfunction has of seeking and obtaining proper help. George Ryan's book is an extremely comprehensive review of male sexual dysfunction. Written by a layman for laymen, it accomplishes its stated purpose—to educate the reader about the problem from which he suffers, and does so in a very readable manner.

If a man believes that nothing can be done about his erection problem, this book should change his mind. This book could be a valuable source of information about his condition—and suggest ways in which he can approach his family doctor on the subject. From these pages, his wife or sexual partner can gain insight into the male viewpoint of the problem. Before seeing a urologist, a man can read about the tests he will undergo and preview options that will be offered him or that he can suggest to the specialist.

Therapy of erectile dysfunction is entering a time of extremely rapid development and change. One must realize that until the early 1960s, the only available treatments were administered by psychiatrists. The psychiatric literature suggested that 95 percent of erectile dysfunction was based on reversible psychological etiology and that the problem could be cured with properly administered time and analysis. It is widely accepted today that the majority of men over the age of 50 with erectile dysfunction have the problem as a result of permanent changes caused by the ravages of hypertension and athersclerosis, diabetes, medication, and the aging process itself.

Although oral agents have been sought to induce erection, existing drugs (most notably yohimbine) have not been shown to be more effective than placebo.

Viagra, from Pfizer Corp., an agent now in the testing phase, but not generally available in the United States, has been shown to be effective, particularly in men with psychogenic or minimal organic disease. Its method of action is to prolong the action of cyclic AMP, the body's own inducer of penile smooth muscle relaxation.

The *most* recent research has shown the importance of ion channels on the surface of penile smooth muscle cells. Two ion channels of particular significance are calcium and potassium. Simply speaking, calcium ion is responsible for smooth muscle contraction (i.e., penile flaccidity) and potassium ion is responsible for smooth muscle relaxation (i.e., erection). Alteration of those two ions represents important venues of future research. Medications that alter the rate of flow of potassium out of cells, known as potassium channel agonists, potentially represent an extremely potent method of causing an erection. A way to introduce these medications into the penis has to be developed, but potassium channel agonists are clearly the next wave of medications in erectile failure therapy.

Perhaps the most exciting therapies on the horizon delve into molecular biology and gene therapy. Animal studies have already been conducted in which genes have been introduced into the penile smooth muscle cells involved in erectile ability. In the future, the potential exists for introduction, perhaps only a few times a year, of those genes into the penis of men suffering from diabetes or anxiety states to allow normalization of function.

In only thirty years, the method of treating men with the demoralizing problem of erectile dysfunction has moved from the analyst's couch to the molecular biologist's gene bank. The next ten years will certainly be witness to truly dramatic developments in this important medical field.

But men with erection problems need not wait for this promising future. They can act without delay to restore their sexual functioning. This book is a valuable guide to the options available to them today.

— ARNOLD MELMAN, M.D.
Professor and Chairman
Department of Urology
Montefiore Medical Center/
    Albert Einstein College of Medicine
Bronx, NY
September 1996

Why You Need to Think for Yourself

The first time a man suffers an episode of impotence, his natural reaction is shame or embarrassment. This is likely to be followed by anger—at himself or his sexual partner, or both. With such feelings, it's difficult for him to think clearly enough to discover what might have caused his impotence in the first place.

His first sexual failure may be just a passing phase, and after a short time he regains his potency without knowing why. But now a doubt has been planted in his mind. He can no longer take his sexuality for granted. And this, in turn, may combine with the original problem and lead to new problems later on. For this reason, it's better to look closely at the problem when it first occurs, instead of hoping it will go away and not come back again.

There's also another reason to act immediately. Impotence can be the first symptom of something else that is happening in the body. For example, it can be a forewarning of cardiac trouble. Take care of the other trouble, and chances are the symptom of impotence will disappear of its own accord.

Denial of the symptom is the easy way out, and the one chosen by many men. The problem with denial is that it won't help a man get an erection again. For his own pride and peace of mind, a man needs to know what is wrong. But male sexual vitality is an emotional minefield. Many men suspect that ignorance is the best policy. Thus, many are big losers, because their problems are often minor and easily treated. If they had chosen to think for themselves, many need not even have had to go to a doctor.

In this book, you will almost certainly find things that fit very closely with things in your own life. Some of these things will be risk factors associated with impotence. If you can change some of these risk factors to lower your overall risk of impotence, you may be on your way to returning as a major performer again.

There are many things that you can do for yourself. After you have done at least some of them, you may need a physician's help if your problem persists. After reading this book, you won't feel dumb and helpless in a doctor's office.

Apart from lab and other test results, a doctor relies on *your* account to a great extent in order to recommend a cure. For example, a doctor writing a prescription for antibiotics for an infected wound does not really need your account of what happened. He can rely on visible symptoms. Although the symptom of impotence is highly visible, its causes are usually invisible to a doctor. Some piece of information from his patient could be crucial to his diagnosis. If the patient has been too panicky to think much about what has caused his impotence, this presents an even greater mystery to the deductive powers of the physician.

If you want to help yourself, you can't escape thinking about the causes of your problem. And by thinking about the causes with the aid of this book, you can save yourself a lot of time, money, and misunderstanding.

The first part of the book describes the various causes of impotence. In these chapters, we see what the risk factors for impotence really are, how they can combine with one another, and how we fall victim to them.

The book's second part gives an account of things that you can do yourself, at work or in your free time, to combat risk factors and regain sexual vitality. Making moderate changes in how a man lives can be enough to restore his full prowess.

In the third part, we look at the help doctors can provide you. We discuss a visit to your regular doctor, and tell you what to expect if you see a urologist. Nearly all cases of impotence can be cured.

These days, almost no man is condemned to impotence, if he is willing to seek a cure. And impotence is no longer viewed as a natural part of the aging process! Between the ages of 20 and 80, the state of a man's health has more influence on his potency than his age. A 30-year-old in bad health is more likely to be impotent than a 70-year-old in good health!

At least 80 percent of the causes of impotence turn out to be physical rather than emotional or psychological. Impotence is not all in the mind. But doing something about it is.

The purpose of this book is simply to present a number of options to you that you may not have thought about. This book is not a definitive account or a comprehensive treatment of the subject. I am neither qualified nor knowledgeable enough to attempt anything of the sort. It's a collection of contemporary reports on what is happening today concerning impotence, and the account dips into all kinds of sources, from technical medical publications, such as the *Journal of Urology*, to newspapers, such as the *Wall Street Journal*, to popular magazines, such as *Men's Health*. There's probably something here for just about everybody to disagree with. But almost certainly, too, there is information here that will be new to you—and possibly of great value.

PART I

HOW THINGS GO WRONG

1

What Men
Don't Talk About

At least 10 million American men suffer from impotence, and the number may be as high as 20 million. If men with partial impotence are included, that number increases to 30 million, according to a National Institutes of Health (NIH) panel on impotence. Comparatively little is known about the incidence of this condition, because men are reluctant to talk about having it. Their unwillingness to discuss the problem leaves many such men feeling emotionally isolated—and can deprive them of a cure. They remain unaware of the fact that most cases of impotence can be cured. Having been brought up to believe that impotence is all in the mind, they don't realize how medical opinion has changed. They don't know that doctors today are more likely to regard impotence as a symptom of a physical medical condition than as an independent mental state. Once the medical condition is cured or alleviated, the symptom of impotence is likely to disappear or at least be diminished.

When researchers of geriatrics took a close look at the healthy aging process, they could find no compelling reasons to include impotence in it. In the absence of disease, there is no reason why an elderly man should not have an erection and satisfying climax. But once he has a medical condition, a male adult of any age has a greatly increased likelihood of impotency.

The good news then is that impotence is more often related to curable physical conditions than psychological ones, and that it is not part of the natural aging process. Everything we do to restore or maintain our good health is likely to be beneficial to our manhood. There's a lot that we can do.

The first part of this book describes the causes of impotence. We first look at a normally functioning male system in Chapter 2. Here you can expect to find answers to questions about the average healthy man. In Chapters 3 and 4, we review impotence risk factors. Some risk factors are direct causes of impotence, while others are indirect; some are predictable, and others are less so. Chapter 3 lists the six illnesses most often associated with impotence, and mentions the brand names of medications that have sexual dysfunction as a side effect. Some of these brands are the best known products in the marketplace.

How many impotence risk factors are in your life? Which ones can you get rid of or avoid completely? Which ones are you stuck with? Can you reduce or manage these? The aim of this book is to help you identify these risk factors and then neutralize or manage them. By doing this, you can lower your likelihood of impotence—or reverse the condition and reclaim sexual potency.

The second part of the book shows you how to combat risk factors and lead a healthier, more potent life. Those illnesses that can't be cured can often be alleviated to the point where their effects in the bedroom are much reduced. These chapters concentrate on things you can do yourself, without professional help. In Chapter 5, after looking at recent mind-body concepts, we show how stress can be thought of as a three-step process and can be mediated at any of these steps. Leading a sedentary life is a risk factor to your health. Chapter 6 suggests things to do about it.

Many men swear by aphrodisiacs, herbs, vitamins, supplements, and over-the-counter remedies. We make no claims for them, but tell you what they are. We also present the latest news on drugs for impotence. Chapters 10 and 11 suggest

many ways you yourself can combat particular impotence
risk factors.

While leading a more healthy lifestyle, some men may still
need to consult a physician. In the third part of the book, we
discuss how to go about finding a specialist in impotence and
benefit from his experience and skilled advice. Should psychotherapy be needed, we look at what you can expect to be
asked on an initial visit to a psychiatrist—and why he's asking
those questions. We hear about the new Caverject injections
and about vacuum devices and penile implants. An end section list phone numbers and addresses where you can get help
for a wide array of problems.

Remember one thing while reading this book: Impotence
can almost always be successfully treated.

PAUL

Paul was 68 and retired for three years when his wife died,
after a brief illness. He stayed with his son and daughter-in-
law in Arizona for a couple of months and then returned home
to Michigan to pick up the threads of his life again. On his
own, he found it more difficult to ignore his erection problem. He could rarely get hard enough to achieve penetration.
His wife had been very patient and loving with him. Any successful erection he had managed at all in the past five years
had been due to her. Now she was gone.

Feeling depressed and lonely, Paul grieved for his dead wife,
slept a lot, and watched old movies on television. Sometimes
he did not leave the house for days. Then he'd pull himself
together and go to see friends, who often introduced him to
desirable women. He always phoned these women afterward
and lunched with them or took them for a drive along the
lakeshore. But he never saw any of them at night or invited
them to his home. What if he couldn't get rid of them? Suppose they wanted to make love and he couldn't satisfy them!
The odds were at least ten to one he couldn't, and he'd be left

feeling ashamed and unmanly. He didn't need a reputation for this among the women of the community.

After three years, he wasn't seeing people much anymore. Paul felt he didn't have much to say to them. He never mentioned a word to anyone about his problem, not even the local doctor. In good weather, he spent his days fishing from a small boat on the big lake. He was getting used to solitude.

The following winter, he was feeling poorly, but never complained. When he didn't feel well enough to go out in the bitter cold, he didn't like to bother anybody by asking for help. He would have died of pneumonia had the mailman not needed a signature on a registered letter and peered in the window when Paul didn't answer the door. The doctor at the local hospital said Paul was also suffering from malnutrition. Since Paul had no financial problems and lived near the town stores, the doctor decided the explanation for his malnutrition was probably depression.

When his son arrived, he told Paul he ought to come live in Arizona or move to a home where he could be cared for. Paul saw his independence threatened and had a talk with the doctor. The doctor sent him to see a urologist in the nearest city. Before the lake ice melted, Paul was seeing a woman regularly. When his son visited again in summer, he was incredulous. He claimed his father looked ten years younger than he had in the previous winter.

IS THERE A MALE MENOPAUSE?

A rapid drop in secretion of the female hormone estrogen causes women to experience menopause at midlife. Although risks and disagreements exist, many women find that estrogen therapy alleviates the unpleasant symptoms of menopause, both physical and emotional. Since men begin to undergo a drop in levels of the male hormone testosterone in their late forties and early fifties, some questions naturally arise. Is there a male menopause at midlife in which sexual potency is, to some extent, lost? And if there is a male menopause, would testosterone therapy relieve this symptom?

Because menopause means the end of menstruation, the terms *andropause* and *viripause* have been suggested for the male process. Called by any name, it is undeniable that most men experience a drop in their testosterone levels of 30 to 40 percent between the ages of 48 and 70.

Dr. S. Mitchell Harman, of the National Institutes of Health, told *Men's Fitness* magazine, when asked if there is a male menopause, that the answer is yes and no. No, because men do not usually experience the sudden drop in hormone levels that women do. Yes, because many men do have a gradual decline in testosterone levels. But he pointed out that testosterone dropped to danger levels only in the rarest cases.

Most men secrete much more testosterone than they ever need for sexual activity, and even when levels drop by 30 or 40 percent over the years, they still have more than enough testosterone for normal functioning. But even when men have almost zero levels of testosterone, they can still have erections and normal sex. Researchers have not been able to directly link testosterone with impotence problems.

In adolescents, testosterone is associated with development of the genitals and also of male secondary sexual characteristics, such as deepening of the voice, muscle development, and facial and body hair. The role of testosterone in male dominance and male sexual desire is widely assumed, but little is known for certain. An adult man who has a gradual drop in his testosterone level may also have a decrease in bone density and an increase in body fat. Meanwhile, too much testosterone has been associated with antisocial behavior, acne, and prostate, heart, and liver problems.

While men do not have a hormone-driven change of life like women, this does not mean that they don't have a midlife crisis. As the body ages physically, it no longer has the vigor and fast recovery time of youth. And in a youth-glorifying culture such as ours, showing almost any signs of aging can cause a man to be labeled as "over the hill." It's only natural to have anxieties about passing from youth to maturity, as it is in experiencing any major change. The transition period may be brief or extended, and it may be hardly noticeable or distressful. In any case, it seems to have little to do with testosterone levels.

WHEN TO BE CONCERNED

Men often wait for years before doing anything about their impotence. When they finally do something about it and are successful, they wonder why they wasted so much time. However, the onset of impotence is often insidious, and it can be difficult for a man to recall exactly when he went from having "problems" to becoming nonfunctional. Denial is one of the ways we cope with stress, and it no doubt plays a role. But the onset of impotence may be so gradual, and interrupted by seeming partial recoveries, men are not alerted to what is happening to them.

As men get older, it usually takes longer for them to achieve an erection. This is normal and needs to be accepted as part of aging. Older men also take longer to achieve another erection after ejaculating. It may take a teenager only a few minutes. Some older men may need twenty-four hours. This is a matter of the normal functioning of a man's body, and no two men are alike. It has nothing to do with impotence.

According to Dr. Steven Morganstern, of the Morganstern Urology Clinic in Atlanta, the number of failures to achieve erection can be indicative of trouble along the following lines:

1 out of 10 encounters	Little reason for immediate concern
1 out of 4 encounters	Strong possibility of chronic impotence
1 out of 2 encounters	Strong evidence that chronic impotence exists

Going from a 1-in-10 to a 1-in-2 failure rate may take from two to five years. Also, it can be easy for a man to kid himself that he's not slowly sliding from 1 in 10 to 1 in 2. There are a thousand ways of blocking out bad news. And hope springs eternal. It's a pity when this happens, because the sooner a man starts to work on this symptom, the easier its solution is.

Dr. Morganstern mentions five early warning signs:

1. *Much fewer morning erections.* As men get older, the urgency and firmness of their erections on awakening gradually lessen. This is normal. However, any fast decline in morning erections may be a symptom of trouble. (Men recovering from surgery or illness may notice an absence of morning erections. They normally return as physical recovery progresses.)

2. *Much fewer spontaneous erections.* When men who get hard easily on seeing an alluring woman or erotic videos notice this doesn't happen anymore, they should regard this as a sign of possible trouble.

3. *Much slower achievement of erection.* With increasing age, men need more stimulation to achieve an erection. A significant increase in this need over a short time may be indicative of a problem.

4. *Increasing inability to assume sexual positions.* When a man accustomed to more variety than the missionary position develops difficulty in achieving positions, he should regard this as a strong warning of approaching trouble.

5. *Increasing inability to maintain an erection.* When a man loses his erection after just a few thrusts, a diversion of arterial blood may be to blame. A narrowing of the iliac arteries may be responsible for the diversion. When a man can't maintain a firm erection for an extended period (about ten minutes), either a leak of venous blood or a diversion of arterial blood may be the cause. The arterial and venous blood mechanics of the penis are a frequent cause of impotence; they are discussed in Chapter 2.

WHAT IMPOTENCE IS AND IS NOT

Impotence can be defined as a man's failure to achieve an erection, or maintain one until the completion of the sexual act. The failure may be partial or complete, and persistent or recurrent. Many men suffer from occasional sexual failure, particularly when physically fatigued or emotionally stressed, but this is normal and should not be viewed as impotence. The medical term for impotence is male erectile disorder.

Having a low sperm count is not the same as being impotent. In fact, a man with a zero sperm count can have erections, orgasms, and a totally satisfying sex life. The number of sperm in the seminal fluid varies greatly from person to person and may be influenced by genetic traits, testicle size, or perhaps even geographic region. Tight jockey shorts or athletic supporters do not decrease sperm counts, as is widely believed. Only a very high fever or very frequent saunas could lower a man's sperm count, and then only temporarily. Cigarettes, street drugs, and alcohol do lower the count. Reports that men today generally have lower sperm counts than those of previous generations have been contradicted by studies pointing out that the opposite may be true! In any case, sperm count has nothing directly to do with ability to achieve an erection.

Premature ejaculation should also not be confused with impotence. In this condition, a man ejaculates with minimal sexual stimulation or before, upon, or shortly after penetration. But so long as he can achieve an erection, he is not impotent. At the other end of the spectrum, inability to achieve an orgasm during intercourse does not involve an erection problem.

Lack of sexual desire on a man's part need not mean that he is incapable of an erection. This is also true for men with an aversion to genital sexual contact. However, if someone lacks a sense of excitement or pleasure during sexual activity, this can be an essential part of his impotence problem.

RESULTS OF STUDIES

The 1985 National Ambulatory Medical Care Survey indicated that impotence was responsible for about 525,000 outpatient visits to physicians. The 1985 National Hospital Discharge Survey estimated that more than 30,000 hospital admissions were for impotence.

The Massachusetts Male Aging Study was conducted between 1987 and 1989. The biggest ever scientific survey of health and aging in American men (aged 40–70), it found that more than half of them (657 out of 1,290) were impotent to some degree. Of the 52 percent of men who suffered from impotence, 17 percent were minimally impotent, 25 percent were moderately impotent, and 10 percent were completely impotent.

In their 1979 reanalysis of A. C. Kinsey's 1948 data, P. H. Gebhard and A. B. Johnson reported that in a sample of 5,460 white males and 177 black males aged 15 through 81 plus, 42 percent had impotence problems.

In other studies in the late 1970s, 40 percent of married men in their thirties said they had erection problems.

WHAT HAS AGE TO DO WITH IMPOTENCE?

The first comprehensive study of male sexual behavior in America was conducted by A. C. Kinsey, of later *Kinsey Report* fame, and published in 1948. In this study of 12,000 men, Kinsey found that impotence increased with age in the following way:

Less than 1 percent before age 19

Less than 3 percent before age 45

6.7 percent between ages 45–55

25 percent by age of 75

In 1986, the Baltimore Longitudinal Study of Aging noted that, by the age of 55, impotence had become a problem for 8 percent of healthy men. For older men with impotence problems, the study gave the following numbers:

25 percent of men by age 65

55 percent of men by age 75

75 percent of men by age 80

In 1992, the Charleston Heart Study Cohort reported that 30 percent of men aged 66–69 were sexually inactive, and 60 percent of men aged 80 or older.

But these statistics need never apply to the individual. And the averages often conceal as much as they reveal. In looking at the numbers, we need to keep in mind that individual differences between men begin to *increase* in late middle age. These differences include organ function. Only in late old age do individual differences decrease and men begin to resemble one another in bodily and other functions. This lack of similarity between individuals is further complicated by the presence or absence of chronic illnesses. With time, few of us escape some kind of chronic ailments, and their influence adds to our individual physical peculiarities. Like our fingerprints, our lives are utterly unique.

Because of these differences and for other reasons, most experts in the field do not attempt to describe an average or normal aging process. Instead, they look at *successful* aging. Looking at successful aging, they then have to decide whether certain things must be accepted as a natural part of the ongoing process or be corrected as undesirable. Impotence belongs firmly in the latter category.

But some deterioration of physical function is a natural part of aging, and as such, it needs to be accepted—but never overestimated! As far as male sexual performance is concerned, the changes take place in four physical domains: the cardiovascular system, the nervous system, hormone levels, and connective body fibers.

Between ages 20 and 80, cardiac output decreases about 1 percent a year. This means that the blood inflow to the penis is a little weaker with every passing year. Additionally, the resistance to blood circulation in organs distant to the heart increases by 1 percent a year after age 40, although this is highly variable. We are talking here about normal changes with aging in healthy men. Illness can greatly speed or magnify these natural changes and their effects.

Concerning the nervous system, the sense of touch decreases with age. Delays at nerve synapses cause messages to take longer being processed by the central nervous system. Neurotransmitter levels may be lower. Sleep disturbances increase with age, and fatigue and irritability resulting from lack of sleep may interfere with male physical functions.

Levels of the male hormone testosterone begin to decrease before middle age, and fibrous tissue in the intertubular spaces of the testicles increases. Lower male hormone levels may result in lower sexual desire.

With age, elastin and other connective body fibers are progressively replaced by less elastic collagen. This may affect the framework of the smooth muscle in the penis.

In the absence of illness or some other contributing factor, it seems hard to find a way that aging itself directly causes impotence. With increasing age, of course, we are more likely to have illnesses and perhaps be more vulnerable to other risk factors. But that's not the same thing. We can't avoid aging, but with care we can avoid some of the negative things associated with it. In other words, it may be within our control whether we remain potent or not.

A study at a Veterans' Administration (VA) hospital vividly showed how impotence was more related to state of health than age. In two groups of patients with similar illnesses, the rate of impotence of the younger group (26 percent) was almost the same as that (27 percent) of the older group aged 65–75.

From a male sexual viewpoint, then, we need to be more concerned with the state of our general health than with our age.

SEXUAL EXPECTATIONS

The NIH panel on impotence found that sexual satisfaction is much affected by sexual expectation. When a man and his sexual partner perceive changes in performance as a consequence of the aging process, they may modify their behavior to accommodate the changes and thereby maintain their sexual satisfaction. In other words, they lower their expectations and thereby avoid disappointment.

Until quite recently, impotence was accepted by both men and women as part of the natural aging process. Except in a few lucky individuals, it was often seen as something to be generally expected, like wrinkles and gray hair. But now men increasingly do not accept impotence as a part of natural aging, and doctors regard a patient's level of expectation as an important indicator of positive attitude.

If a man's level of expectations are unreasonably high, he's placing stress on himself and is bound to feel some distress. On the other hand, a man may too easily accept potency problems as a part of aging and give in without a fight. When the Massachusetts study mentioned earlier found that men suffered relatively little sexual dissatisfaction with aging because their expectations were so low, you have to wonder if they weren't all going too gently into that good night.

What are reasonable expectations? Conventional wisdom has it that a man's sex drive peaks at around the age of 18 and that it's all downhill from that point on, with the downhill slope becoming progressively and alarmingly steeper from the forties onward. While it's undeniable that aging brings changes to every man's sexual life, it's equally undeniable that plenty of men enjoy a healthy and active sex life through their fifties, sixties, and seventies—and even into their eighties! In spite of continuing good health, all men have to accept some loss in their sensitivity to touch and in the tone of their penile smooth muscle.

What other strictly age-related factor is there? Some therapists believe that older man find it harder to have an erection

based solely on fantasy. This loss of imaginative ability may or
may not correlate with age. One therapist suggested that when
a man loses some of his ability to fantasize, he should have no
trouble making up for it at bookstores, magazine stands, and
video stores.

CHECKPOINT

- Impotence can almost always be successfully treated.
- Impotence much more often has a physical cause than a
  psychological cause. It's not all in the mind.
- Don't try to see things through on your own. No man is an
  island.
- There's nothing you can tell a doctor about sexual
  problems that he hasn't heard before—or perhaps
  suffered from himself!
- Male hormone levels are almost certainly not the prob-
  lem, nor is sperm count.
- Seek advice when you notice early warning signs.
- Impotence plays no part in successful aging.
- Sexually, men need to be more concerned with the state
  of their general health than with their age.

2

The Functioning
Male System

The purpose of having an erection is for the penis to penetrate the vagina. While it is possible to have an ejaculation without an erection, most of the pleasurable sensations are lost and, from a biological viewpoint, the sperm is less likely to find its way to an egg.

The mechanism of an erection is often compared to a car's hydraulic brake system. By pressing on the brake pedal, you exert pressure on fluid in a confined area and the fluid presses against its boundaries. In human erections, relaxation of smooth muscle allows blood to rush into the penis faster than it can flow out again, and the pressure buildup inside the penis causes it to become erect.

HOW THE PENIS BECOMES ERECT

You need to know very little anatomy to understand the mechanical details of an erection. The erectile tissue of the penis consists of two paired corpora cavernosa and a corpus spongiosum. The corpus spongiosum surrounds the urethra (through which, at different times, semen and urine exit) and forms the glans or head of the penis. The two corpora cavernosa are cylinders that run lengthwise inside the penis. Each is enclosed in a thick fibrous sheath and is filled with spongelike tissue with numerous interconnected spaces. The spaces are lined by tissue with a rich blood supply. The walls of these spaces are formed of smooth muscle and an expandable frame consisting of elastin, fibroblasts, and collagen. When the penis is flaccid, the spaces in the erectile tissue are empty. Blood is prevented from flowing into them by smooth muscle whose normal state is contraction.

As an erection begins, arterial blood flows to the two corpora cavernosa through the right and left cavernosal arteries. Many corkscrew-shaped arteries, with muscular walls, branch off each cavernosal artery and open directly into the spaces of the spongelike tissue.

Blood leaves the corpora cavernosa through small veins located between the periphery of the spongelike tissue and the fibrous sheath. These small veins flow into larger ones that pierce the sheath.

Nerves connect the spinal cord to the penis. They run from the thoracic, lumbar, and sacral segments of the spinal cord, all in the lower back. The pudendal nerve connects the penis with nerve fibers running to the skin of the penis and genital area.

Erections are initiated by nerve messages, which in turn originate from genital sensory stimuli or from brain stimuli. Both kinds of stimuli probably act synergistically. Much is known about the nerve pathways of sensory stimuli, but the pathways of stimuli inside and from the brain are much less well understood. The stimuli seem to be integrated in the brain's hypothalamus, and from there they travel as a message down the spinal cord.

The message delivered by nerves to smooth muscle in the penis is not to become stiff but to relax. The muscular walls of the arteries are told to dilate. Blood rushes through the widened cavernosal and corkscrew-shaped arteries into the spaces of the spongelike tissue inside the corpora cavernosa. Their smooth-muscle walls relaxed, these spaces swell with blood. The blood system's pressure causes engorgement of the spongelike tissue and makes it swell against the enclosing fibrous sheath.

The small veins that would normally drain this blood are compressed between the swollen spongelike tissue and the fibrous sheath. This cuts off the escape route of the blood. Pressure builds. The penis becomes rigid. As long as inflow is maintained and outflow is prevented, the blood's pressure inside the corpora cavernosa causes the erection to continue.

Detumescence takes place when the smooth-muscle walls of the spongelike spaces and corkscrew arteries contract. A nerve message causes them to do this, and decreased blood inflow and collapse of the spaces result. In turn, the compression on the small veins is eased and they begin to drain off blood. As the process continues, the penis becomes flaccid.

From this, we can say that there are four physiological requirements for a penis to become erect: (1) intact nerve connections, (2) intact arterial supply, (3) appropriately responsive smooth muscle in the corpora cavernosa, and (4) intact venous mechanics.

ROLE OF NEUROTRANSMITTERS

A nerve cell has long extensions that extend toward similar extensions of other nerve cells. They form an incredibly complex network in the brain and act as highways for the brain's messages to and from the body. Messages are carried along nerve cells electrically. In the gap between two nerve extensions, the message may be carried from one nerve cell to another either electrically or chemically.

Electrical communication across the gap is much faster than chemical. Electrical communication is what permits cats, for example, to have such fast physical reactions to things around them. Humans depend more on chemical communication across the gap. But why would evolution favor a slower means of communication? Surely fast reactions mean everything. Apparently not in all situations. We can easily understand how lightning-fast instinctive reactions to fixed patterns of situations could be benefical to a hunting carnivore like a cat. But what the cat gains in speed, it loses in flexibility. Cats react before they have time to consider options. Humans, with slower chemical communication across nerve gaps, have greater flexibility and adaptability. They have time to think.

The chemicals that carry messages across the gap between nerve cells are known as neurotransmitters and neuropeptides. One nerve ending releases the chemical, and it is picked up by another nerve ending in receptors specially designed to accept that chemical. The nerve ending that releases the chemical into the gap may reabsorb that chemical and thereby reduce its concentration in the gap. This is referred to as reuptake. Many mood-altering drugs—licit and illicit—work by interfering in some way with this chemical transmission of messages.

Neurotransmitters involved in the mechanism of erections may be affected by intentional and unintentional reactions with various drugs. Comparatively little is known about neurotransmitters in general.

Dilation of the cavernosal arteries of the penis has been studied only in animals and seems to be due to a nonadrenergic, noncholinergic neurotransmitter. The contraction of these arteries in humans, which causes detumescence, has been shown to be controlled by adrenergic nerves through alpha-adrenergic receptors. Nerves containing vasoactive intestinal polypeptide (VIP) and neuropeptide Y are known to be associated with the cavernosal and corkscrew arteries.

The smooth muscle around the cavities in spongelike tissue relaxes under the influence of cholinergic and nonadrenergic, noncholinergic neurotransmitters—perhaps VIP—resulting in an erection. This smooth muscle contracts when adrenergic nerves release norepinephrine into the nerve gaps and it is taken up by alpha1-adrenergic receptors. Cholinergic nerves seem to modulate both the relaxation and contraction processes rather than act directly.

As mentioned, the cells lining the spaces in the spongelike tissue have a rich blood supply. They cause the smooth muscle upon which they rest to relax or contract by releasing substances carried by the bloodstream. These substances include prostaglandins, endothelium-derived relaxing factor (thought to be nitric oxide or a similar molecule), endothelium-derived hyperpolarizing factor, and the peptide endothelin.

To put it briefly, when these neurotransmitters or chemical messengers tell the penile smooth muscle to relax and the cavernosal arteries to dilate, a man has an erection. When something interferes with or blocks that message, or when the message is not sent at all, there is a reason for it. Finding that reason, if possible, is a logical way of going about making a change.

Prescribed medications and street drugs are responsible for many cases of impotence, probably mostly through their effect on neurotransmitters.

ORGASM

Formed in the testes, sperm travel to the epididymis, a mass of tubules at the back of the testes, where they stay for about twenty-four hours. The sperm then move to the vas deferens, a tube about two feet long, in which they may be stored and remain viable for about a month. (This tube is cut in a vasectomy, rendering the male voluntarily sterile. This does not cause impotence.)

During sexual stimulation, the nerves cause the urethral and bulbourethral glands to secrete mucus. During intercourse, this mucus flows through the urethra as lubrication, although most of this is supplied by the female sex organs. When the sexual stimulation becomes very intense, nerves initiate the process of emission, which is the forerunner of ejaculation. Emission is thought to begin with the contraction of the vas deferens, which forces sperm into the internal opening of the urethra. Then contractions of the prostate gland and seminal

vesicles force prostatic fluid and seminal fluid into the urethra, where they mix together and with the sperm and mucus
as they move onward.

Further nerve signals cause rhythmic contractions of the
internal genital organs and contraction of muscles that put
pressure on the corpora cavernosa. These in turn cause rhythmic, wavelike increases in pressure along the urethra, resulting in ejaculation of the semen. Rhythmic movements of the
pelvic muscles thrust the penis forward and cause the semen
to be ejaculated deep in the vagina.

The processes of emission and ejaculation together make up
the male orgasm. Once ejaculation takes place, sexual excitement quickly almost disappears and the penis becomes flaccid.

Many men complain that intercourse and orgasm become less
satisfying as they grow older. Declining tactile sensitivity and
declining tone of their penile smooth muscle may account for
a diminished climax, according to William H. Masters, M.D.,
Virginia E. Johnson, and Robert C. Kolodny, M.D., in *Heterosexuality*. Additionally, older men produce less semen, which
lessens the sense of release.

But Robert O. Hawkins Jr., Ph.D., a professor of health sciences at the State University of New York at Stony Brook, disagrees. "The standard belief is that older men need more stimulation to achieve the same level of sexual response," he told
Glamour magazine. "But I think it's less of a problem of physical aging than of life pressures. Older men need more time to
get the rest of the world out of their head."

A 29-year-old man agreed with Hawkins. He told *Glamour*,
"In college it didn't matter how big a test you had the next
day—sex was more important. Now any insignificant problem at the office is right there in bed with us."

He and others claimed that foreplay had definitely helped
reduce their stress levels.

To make the orgasm itself more enjoyable, San Francisco
sex therapist Louanne Cole, Ph.D., recommends the "balk

method." In the April 1996 issue of *Men's Fitness*, she explained that the balk method means going into the windup but not throwing the pitch. A man approaches the point of no return but stops just short of it. To do this, he needs to change his pace when he is close to orgasm, regain full control, and work his way to that point again. Doing this several times will allow him, finally, to climax longer and more intensely.

THE PROSTATE GLAND

It needs to be said from the outset that swelling of the prostate gland does not cause impotence. Surgery and drugs for prostate cancer can cause impotence, and a prostate infection might make intercourse painful.

The prostate is a walnut-sized gland (really a group of glands) situated under the bladder. It is close to the urethra, the tube that carries semen and urine through the penis. Thus enlargement or infection of the prostate can interfere with urination. Because the prostate is close to the front wall of the rectum, a physician can test its condition with a finger. The prostate secretes fluid into the urethra, supplying about half the seminal fluid in which the sperm move. The gland has no other known function.

The seminal vesicles supply the the other half of the seminal fluid, and these fluids, together with the sperm, are known as semen. When the prostate is surgically removed, the ejaculatory fluid is lost—but this does not involve any major loss of pleasurable sensation on ejaculation, provided that certain nerves are not severed.

The prostate is a well-known health hazard for men. Its three major disorders are benign enlargement, prostatitis, and cancer.

Benign prostatic enlargement. When the prostate enlarges, it may press on the urethra and narrow the passageway for urine. The symptoms of this condition—known also as benign prostatic hyperplasia—are difficulty in starting to urinate, a lessened force of the urine stream, and a dribbling of urine after urination is finished. The onset of these symptoms is usually gradual. Advanced cases may result in blockage of the urethra and backup of urine, which is an emergency medical condition.

At the age of 40, about 10 percent of men have some enlargement of the prostate; by the age of 60, almost all men do. The prostate may enlarge because of hormonal changes with aging, but no cause is known for sure. Benign enlargement means enlargement not due to cancer, and is usually caused by overgrowth of urethral glands in the interior of the prostate.

Surgery to relieve blockage of urine flow is of several kinds. A transurethral incision is an outpatient procedure in which a flexible endoscope is passed through the urethra to make small pressure-lessening cuts in the prostate. For more advanced swelling, a transurethral resection may be necessary, but this procedure carries a 5–20 percent risk of impotence. A more recent technique, transurethral ultrasound-guided laser-induced prostatectomy, is believed to be more precise and thus less damaging, but is still in its proving phase.

The drug finasteride (Proscar) was thought to be effective in reducing benign prostate enlargement. In an unusual comparative study, however, the drug terazosin (Hytrin) was compared with Proscar. Hytrin was found to be effective in the treatment of an enlarged prostrate gland, but Proscar was found to be no better than the dummy pills used as a control in the tests. The year-long study on 1,200 men was conducted by a team led by Dr. Herbert Lepor of the Veterans Affairs Medical Center in New York City and New York University. The study was published in the August 22, 1996, issue of the *New England Journal of Medicine*. Both Hytrin and Proscar are approved by the FDA. The rate of impotence associated with Hytrin is 1.6 percent or lower. In an international twelve-month controlled clinical trial of Proscar on 543 men, 3.7 percent of the men became impotent, 3.3 percent suffered a lowered sex drive, and 2.8 percent complained of decreased volume of ejaculate. The drug flutamine (Eulexin) causes a higher rate of impotence, as does estrogen therapy.

In May 1996, the FDA approved the Prostatron, a device that kills excess prostate tissue with microwaves and that has no significant effect on sexual function. A catheter from the Prostatron is inserted into the urethra and pushed into the prostate. Microwaves travel through the catheter to destroy the excess tissue. Dr. John Lynch, urology chief at Georgetown University Medical Center, told the *New York Times* that using the Prostatron is a one-hour, outpatient procedure that works better than drugs and is safer than surgery.

Of 375 men over the age of 45 who underwent the procedure in a study, 75 percent noticed a lessening of symptoms. However, a third of the men were temporarily unable to urinate because of swelling. Dr. David A. Kessler, the commissioner of the Food and Drug Administration (FDA), said that while using the Prostatron was not a cure, it effectively treated the symptoms.

For prevention of prostate enlargement, see Chapter 7.

Prostatitis. According to Harvard Medical School doctors W. I. Bennett, S. E. Goldfinger, and G. T. Johnson, fortunate is the man who makes it through life without at least one bout of prostatitis. An infection of the prostate gland, prostatitis may be either acute or chronic. With acute prostatitis, a man often feels pain at the base of his penis and has painful urination and a fever. A cloudy fluid may drip from the urethra. The bacterial agent can normally be identified through a lab test on a urine sample and the infection cured with antibiotics. When the condition is not caused by a bacterial agent, treatment can be more complex.

Chronic prostatitis consists of recurrent low-grade infections that can cause much discomfort and annoyance. The cause is often difficult to pinpoint. The bacterial agent may be particularly persistent or resistant to antibiotics or of an unusual type. Doctors who believe that there may be an emotional component prescribe tranquilizers. Dr. E. David Crawford, chairman of the division of urology at the University of Colorado Health Sciences Center in Denver, suggested three causes of nonbacterial prostatitis to *Men's Health* magazine: (1) Stress may cause a man to unconsciously clench his bladder sphincter, forcing urine back into the prostate. (Solution: Manage the stress.) (2) Stop-and-go urination can have a similar result. (Solution: Don't stop until you're done.) (3) Dehydration from work or athletic exertion can result in a highly concentrated urine that can inflame the prostate. (Solution: Drink lots of water.)

Infrequent ejaculations, prolonged sitting, and coffee have also been seen as causes or contributory factors, but no agreement exists on this.

For prevention of prostate infection, see Chapter 7.

Prostate cancer. This condition has been the subject of many recent books and has generated much media coverage because of its apparent fast increasing incidence among American men. A *Time* magazine list of prominent men who died of prostate cancer includes rock star Frank Zappa at 52, media executive Steve Ross at 65, actor Telly Savalas at 70, French ex-president Francois Mitterrand (who kept his condition secret for eleven years) at 79, and Iranian Ayatullah Khomeini at 89. *Time's* list of survivors of prostate cancer surgery includes Bob Dole, Sidney Poitier, General Norman Schwarzkopf, Robert Goulet, King Hussein of Jordan, Jesse Helms, Richard Petty, Marion Barry, and Michael Milken. Not long ago, public disclosure about such an intimate condition would have been unthinkable. But, today, if the victor of the Gulf War and the king of stock car racing are willing to talk about their prostates publicly, there's little excuse for a man who hesitates to discuss genital or sexual things with his doctor—or for a doctor who does not dicuss such things with his patients.

Although prostate cancer is one of the leading causes of cancer deaths in men, it generally develops slowly and therefore is not seen as a mortal threat in older men. In fact, most men over 80 probably have slow-growing minor developments of prostate cancer and will almost certainly die of other causes before it can become a threat to them. However, when a man potentially still has many years left to him or if the prostate cancer is more quickly growing, surgical or other intervention is necessary.

Radical prostatectomy, external-beam radiation, "seed" radiation, and cryotherapy all carry a risk of impotence. Hormone therapy often involves a loss of sex drive. A prostatectomy almost invariably causes a man to be impotent if the surgeon cuts two nerve bundles that control erections that run along the surface of the prostate gland. Dr. Patrick Walsh, of the Johns Hopkins Hospital, developed a technique to move the nerve bundles aside before removing the prostate. Walsh says this can be done only when the cancer does not lie close to the nerve bundles. He claims that 90 percent of his patients under 50 who undergo this procedure regain their potency.

Catching the cancer before it has spread beyond the prostate is essential. By the time cancer can be felt in a digital rectal exam, it has often spread into the body. The PSA (prostate-specific antigen) test measures the blood level of an antigen produced by the prostate. When the level rises too high, it indicates probable trouble. But the PSA test has run into difficulties, because benign prostate enlargement, frequently found in older men, also elevates PSA levels. It is claimed that only one in three men with elevated PSA levels who undergo a biopsy turns out to have cancer. In June 1996, Biomerica announced a five-minute PSA test that can be done more cheaply in a doctor's office. The company said it would sell the test, called EZ-PSA, overseas while waiting for FDA clearance to sell it in America.

Finally, a word about scare tactics. The *Time* article on prostate cancer mentioned "epidemic levels in the U.S." and claimed that "1 in 5 American men will develop prostate cancer in his lifetime." Mathematics professor and author John Allen Paulos put these statistics in a more realistic light for the *Wall Street Journal*. In reality, if you are 40, your chance of developing prostate cancer in the next ten years is only one in a thousand. Over the next twenty years after that, it is one chance in a hundred. When you are 70, your chance of getting any kind of cancer, including prostate, is only one in twenty. After age 70, your chances increase dramatically.

Michael Korda's book *Man to Man: Surviving Prostate Cancer* is an engagingly honest first-person account of what it is like to have surgery for prostate cancer. Other sources of information are listed under "Prostate Cancer" in the appendix "Where to Get Help."

For prevention of prostate cancer, see Chapter 7.

PENILE ENLARGEMENT SURGERY

According to a 1996 *Wall Street Journal* article, 10,000 to 15,000 penis-lengthening or -widening surgeries have been performed in the United States since the early 1990s. A man can expect to spend $6,000 to $7,000—and an hour on the table—at a doctor's office rather than a hospital. The procedure is advertised in men's magazines; more than thirty Web sites give information about it; there are toll-free phone numbers to call; and the surgeons accept Visa and MasterCard.

Lengthening the penis does not involve any actual lengthening of the organ itself. The procedure is dependent on the fact that a man's penis extends back into his body. The surgeon severs a ligament that attaches the penis to the pubic bone, and this permits more of its length to extend beyond the body. Claims are made that two inches can be added to its length.

Widening or thickening of the penis is done through a liposuction-like technique—injecting fat from the abdomen or other parts of the body beneath the skin of the penis.

The good news is that men who have previously felt bad about being modestly endowed feel a renewed sex drive and a new confidence in themselves that extends from the bedroom to the boardroom. The bad news is reflected in the high number of lawsuits by men who have undergone the procedure. Whether these bad results—scarring or lumpiness of the penis, impotence, and even death—were due to poor surgical technique or to risks inherent in the procedure is not clear at this stage.

According to the *Wall Street Journal*, the American Urological Association and the American Society for Aesthetic Plastic Surgery both say that phalloplasty, as the surgical procedure is known, has not been shown to be safe or effective. No comprehensive clinical or research studies on penile enlargement have been published. The FDA does not monitor the surgery because no implants or drugs are involved. Since most procedures are performed in doctor's offices or clinics, hospital authorities do not review them. State health authorities respond only to complaints about individual physicians. Malpractice insurers sometimes cover doctors for penis lengthening but rarely for fat-injection widening.

Dr. Gary Rheinschild, a urologist in Anaheim, California, told the *Journal* that he repairs a lot of bungled penile surgery. He also said that he does not use fat injections himself because they often result in concavities, nodules, and asymmetrical-looking penises. He recommended dermal grafts instead. In this procedure, two strips of fat are taken from the gluteal folds (where the thighs meet the buttocks) and are implanted on either side of the penis.

Don't get hustled by ads or media hype into thinking that phalloplasty is low-risk surgery. Insist on finding out about your physician's record of success. And maybe reconsider whether you really need more than you were given.

SOME RELEVANT DATA

The following data were reviewed by Dr. Irwin Goldstein, professor of urology at Boston University School of Medicine, and Dr. Dudley Seth Danoff, attending physician at Cedars Sinai Medical Center in Los Angeles, for an article by Joe Kita in the March 1996 issue of *Men's Health*:

- The average length of an erect penis is 5.1 inches.
- The average length of a flaccid penis is 3.5 inches.
- The longest medically verified erect penis was 12 inches.

- The average number of erections during a night's sleep is five.
- The average duration of each nocturnal erection is 20–30 minutes.
- An erect penis contains 8 to 10 times the amount of blood of a flaccid penis.
- The average length and width of testicles are 1.4 by 1 inch.
- The average man produces 50,000 sperm per minute, or 72 million per day.
- The number of sperm in the average ejaculation is 200 to 600 million.
- An ejaculation containing less than 50 million sperm may mean infertility.
- The average life span of sperm in a woman's body is one to two days.
- The average volume of semen in an ejaculation is 0.5 to 1 teaspoon.
- The average number of spurts in an ejaculation is 3 to 10.
- The farthest medically recorded distance traveled by an ejaculation is 11.7 inches.

CHECKPOINT

- For an erection to take place, four systems need to be in working order: nerve connections, arterial supply, smooth muscle response, and venous mechanics.
- Medications frequently cause impotence, probably by interfering with neurotransmitters.
- A vasectomy is not a physical cause of impotence.
- Swelling of the prostate gland does not cause impotence, although surgery and drugs for it and prostate cancer can be a cause.

3

Illness, Medication, and Impotence

Until fairly recently, impotence was thought to be all in the mind. Today, however, physical illness is regarded as its most frequent cause. One group of doctors claimed that physically ill men are six times more likely to be impotent than healthy men. In this chapter, we look at the six illnesses most often associated with impotence. Using the phrase *associated with* avoids making a claim that the illness is *directly* responsible for the impotence.

Human biology is complex, and simple cause-and-effect relationships are not the rule. Often, a combination of causes is responsible for an effect. Additionally, the susceptibility of the person has to be taken into account. Doctors frequently see patients exposed to similar disease-causing circumstances that some succumb to and some don't. An important factor seems to be whether a person is *vulnerable* to a particular illness. This vulnerability may be a result of the person's genetic makeup and may also be affected by the current state of his or her immune system. Many doctors believe that individuals have their own special vulnerabilities, and that getting to know what they are is a major aspect of personal preventive medicine.

RISK FACTORS

One way that physicians deal with the complex things that contribute to illhealth is to label them risk factors. As such, we can more easily understand and hopefully manage them. For example, if several members of a man's family have died early of, say, heart disease, his family health history must be looked on as a risk factor. Chances are good that his family history indicates his own genetic makeup and a proclivity for heart trouble.

Ilnesses are risk factors, since having one illness can be a risk factor for contracting another. Indicators that are not illnesses themselves can be risk factors, such as family history or having a high cholesterol level. But risk factors exist in lifestyles, too. Not wearing a seat belt in a car is a risk factor. So is drinking too much alcohol. Cigarette smoking is a risk factor for several serious illnesses. Risk factors can be psychological—for example, depression, which is thought to leave people vulnerable to many illnesses.

When we think in terms of risk factors, several interesting concepts emerge. First and foremost is the possibility of the management of risk. We can stop smoking cigarettes and abusing alcohol. We can buckle up and drive safely. There are no guarantees, but such measures do pay off. The most dramatic example of this in public health has been the huge reduction in the death rate of Americans due to heart disease. This has been credited to more people eating a diet lower in fat and getting some exercise.

Another concept is that we are not prisoners of our risk factors. By getting to understand them, we can to some extent free ourselves from them. Consider the man with a family history of heart trouble. He is not condemned to heart trouble himself. He may not have inherited the vulnerabilities of his less fortunate family members, but it would be safer for him to assume that he has and to make provisions for them. Following American Heart Association recommendations on diet would help neutralize these risk factors. With a few other obvious cardiac precautions, such as not smoking, he can dramatically change the odds against him. Changing the odds is what it's all about. When the odds appear to be stacked against you, you can change the rules of the game by changing your behavior.

As said before, physicians don't regard the origin of disease as a simple cause-and-effect sequence. Some doctors have suggested that two or three risk factors need to be present simultaneously. In addition, a trigger factor may be needed. Suppose a man has a family history of heart disease, is a heavy smoker and is overweight. Those are three risk factors. The trigger factor might be a climb up a steep hill or an argument with his wife. On the other hand, he could have all three risk factors, climb and argue a lot, and live to be ninety! But the odds heavily favor one outcome over the other.

Impotence is definitely associated with certain conditions—medical, psychological, and lifestyle. We will regard all these as risk factors. In this chapter and the next, we will look at the known risk factors for impotence. Recognizing them as such will often be enough to suggest ways of managing them.

Age is a risk factor for impotence. But an even greater risk factor is poor health.

MASSACHUSETTS MALE AGING STUDY

At the present state of medical knowledge, physicians cannot trace cause-and-effect linkages of risk factors with scientific certainty. But scientific knowledge is not the prime motivation of a healer. A healer tries first and foremost to cure. Doctors often have to work in the absence of hard science, and it is not for nothing that they refer to the art of medicine. Each physician has his own inborn and learned talents for healing. They rely on clinical studies for medical, as distinct from scientific, information.

In the first chapter, the Massachusetts Male Aging Study (MMAS) was referred to as the biggest ever survey of male sexual health in America. In this chapter and the next, we will refer to its findings on what most frequently causes impotence. The MMAS was a cross-sectional, community-based, random-sample, multidisciplinary epidemiologic survey of health and aging in men 40–70 years old. The study was conducted between 1987 and 1989 in eleven randomly selected cities and towns in the Boston area. Of 1,709 men approached in the study, 1,290 (75.5 percent) provided complete answers to all the questions on sexual function.

The men were asked nine questions about their erectile potency. Additionally, they were asked to rate their potency according to four grades: (1) not impotent, (2) minimally impotent, (3) moderately impotent, and (4) completely impotent.

As mentioned in the first chapter, more than half the men (657 out of 1,290) had some degree of erectile dysfunction. The numbers were as follows:

Minimally impotent	210	17%
Moderately impotent	322	25%
Completely impotent	125	10%
TOTAL	657	52%

The study examined how male sexual activity and expectations changed between the ages of 40 and 70 years. Most of the men showed a steady decline in sexual activity with age. But their sexual satisfaction remained more or less unaffected, because their expectations also declined.

Those who stayed in good health were most likely to be sexually satisfied. Decreased sexual satisfaction was most likely to be found in men who were depressed or angry.

The probability that a 40-year-old man had problems with impotence was 38.9 percent, and a 70-year-old man, 67.1 percent.

THE SIX ILLNESSES
MOST OFTEN ASSOCIATED WITH IMPOTENCE

In the MMAS, the medical conditions most often associated with impotence were heart disease, treated diabetes, high blood pressure, an untreated ulcer, arthritis, and allergy.

At a June 1966 meeting at Rockefeller University, Dr. Adrian Dobs, an endocrinologist who teaches at Johns Hopkins University, said that men should look at declining sexual function as a possible warning of impending disease, particularly heart disease or diabetes.

The very short commentary on these six conditions reflects the lack of medical knowledge on how exactly they are associated with impotence. In particular, it is usually hard to tell whether the medical condition itself is the most important risk factor or the medication being taken for it, or a combination of the two.

Cardiovascular Disease

Cardiovascular disease is the medical illness that most frequently causes impotence. This is readily understandable when you consider that an erection depends on an inflow of arterial blood to the penis. Anything that intereferes with the blood inflow, such as partially blocked arteries, may cause a problem. Men who have had coronary bypass surgery or who suffer from myocardial infarction, stroke, peripheral blood disease, or high blood pressure are most likely to have problems with the supply of arterial blood to the penis. The four greatest risk factors for arterial insufficiency are: high blood pressure, smoking, diabetes, and low HDL.

Dr. Steven Morganstern stresses three arterial problems: hardening and narrowing of arteries, blockage of arteries, and thickening of the blood. Hardening of arteries (arteriosclerosis) refers to the interior of arterial walls becoming lined with fatty deposits over time, like mineral deposits in an old pipe. This can result in two problems: a reduced flow of blood and inability of the penile artery to dilate when called to do so to facilitate an erection. A well-known symptom indicating possible hardening of the arteries is pain in the legs after vigorous walking. See a doctor before forming any conclusions, however.

The interior diameter of penile arteries is very small, and they have little excess capacity. Additionally, some men are born with narrower arteries than others. Substances in cigarette smoke cause the constriction of blood vessels. Radiation therapy of the pelvic area frequently causes scarring that results in the penile arteries losing their ability to dilate.

Blockage of arteries can be a result of surgery, injury, or aging. Surgery on blood vessels in another part of the body may cause a fatty deposit to break loose and be carried by the bloodstream to an artery through which it cannot pass and therefore blocks. Injury in the pelvic region may cause blockage of arteries. With age, men may develop blockages in the major arteries leading to the legs, which can cause them walking problems. Often, these men also have potency problems, because the arteries to the penis are offshoots of those to the legs and suffer blockage as well.

Thickening of the blood and a consequent lack of fluidity can result from sickle-cell anemia or chemotherapy. In the latter case, it may be reversible when the therapy has ended.

Anything that permits a too rapid blood outflow from the penis also interferes with an erection, but this is less common than inflow problems. In a normal erection, the swelling spongelike tissue presses against the fibrous sheath of the corpora cavernosa, thereby compressing the small veins and shutting off their outflow. This is called the corporal venoocclusive mechanism. Venous leakage may occur because of insufficient smooth muscle relaxation. In cases where the smooth muscle relaxes normally, the trouble may be with the fibroelastic framework on which the smooth muscle rests. This framework may no longer be elastic enough to be pressed against the fibrous sheath. The loss of elasticity may be due to age, cross-linking of collagen fibers, or collagen changes caused by low HDL. Injury to the penis from any cause, including surgery and priapism, may also be responsible.

The MMAS found one combination of three risk factors to be strongly associated with impotence. Those three risk factors were: heart disease, high blood pressure, and a low HDL blood level.

In the MMAS, men with treated heart disease were four times more likely to be completely impotent than men without heart disease. Cigarette smoking and treated heart disease were a combination likely to double the likelihood of complete impotence.

Four Vascular Self-Diagnostic Tests

If you think you may have blood-flow problems, you need professional advice. These four home tests are indicators of vascular problems, but not conclusive proof that they exist. They are recommended by Dr. Steven Morganstern.

1. *Vigorous walk test*. Walk briskly for about a mile. Afterward, if you feel pain in either or both of your calves, this may indicate insufficient blood flow.

2. *Cold penis test*. If your penis constantly feels cold, even when the rest of your body feels warm, this may indicate poor arterial supply.

3. *Blue penis test*. A characteristic blue color of the penis indicates impaired arterial supply. This is easier to observe with light skin than with dark.

4. *Penile hard areas test*. These hard areas can typically be felt along both sides of the penis, close to where it emerges from the body. They are deposits in vascular tissue and may cause erection problems by obstructing blood flow. On first noticing them, some men fear they are caused by cancer, which is not the case.

Dr. Morganstern also recommends that while you are performing a genital self-examination, you check your testicles for lumps or swelling that may provide an early warning of cancer.

Diabetes

The MMAS results showed that men with treated diabetes were three times more likely to be completely impotent, and twice as likely to be minimally impotent, than men without diabetes. In other studies, primarily on exclusively diabetic patients, estimates of impotence range from 35–50 percent and up to 75 percent. In 1980, M. Ellenberg found that 50–60 percent of diabetic men have impotence problems.

The age of a diabetic man is relevant, with an increase in the rate of impotence from 15 percent at 30–34 years to 55 percent at 60 years. Regardless of whether a man's diabetes is insulin- or noninsulin-dependent, he is likelier to become impotent at an earlier age than other men, often within ten years of diagnosis of the condition.

While cardiovascular disease is thought to be the medical condition most frequently associated with impotence, this is disputed by some experts, who believe that diabetes deserves this unfortunate title.

Diabetes usually exists in association with other impotence risk factors. It may be accompanied by vascular, high blood pressure, and even nerve damage risk factors. Obesity and alcoholism are frequent. Depression is often an acompanying psychological risk factor.

Doctors, counselors, families, and patients themselves are sometimes unaware that young and middle-aged men with diabetes can develop impotence problems. A lack of willingness to discuss sexual problems can be a roadblock to finding a cure.

High Blood Pressure

In the MMAS, men being treated for high blood pressure were significantly more likely to be completely impotent than men without that condition. High blood pressure (hypertension) is often classified as a cardiovascular disease. Many drugs used to treat high blood pressure have depression as a side effect. The addition of this risk factor doubles the risk of impotence.

Ulcer

In the MMAS, men with an untreated ulcer were almost twice as likely as other men to have impotence problems. Impotence problems caused by anti-ulcer drugs are usually reversible when they stop being used.

Arthritis

In the MMAS, men with untreated arthritis were significantly more likely than other men to have impotence problems. Among men with arthritis, those who smoked were almost twice as likely to be completely impotent as those who didn't.

Allergy

In the MMAS, men with an untreated allergy were significantly more likely than other men to suffer from impotence problems. Additionally, antihistamines for the treatment of allergies are capable of causing potency problems.

MEDICATIONS

Well-known New York physician and author, Isadore Rosenfeld, places medications high on his list of possible causes of impotence. In fact, his rule for virtually any symptom, including impotence, is: When you wonder what's causing it, look into your medicine cabinet first. Back in 1983, M. F. Slag and colleagues reported in the *Journal of the American Medical Association* that among the outpatients of one medical clinic, 25 percent of the cases of impotence were associated with drugs. The NIH panel on impotence found that percentage to hold a decade later. According to Robert J. Krane and his colleagues at the Boston University Medical Center, it is not known precisely how most drugs cause impotence.

In the MMAS, men were significantly more likely to be completely impotent who took certain medications, as shown below.

Medication	*Greater likelihood of complete impotence*
Vasodilators	Almost four times
Cardiac drugs	Almost three times
Hypoglycemic agents	Almost three times
Antihypertensives	Significantly

It came as no surprise that the patterns between men taking cardiac, hypoglycemic, or antihypertensive drugs matched those of men under treatment for cardiovcascular disease, diabetes, or high blood pressure, respectively. Additionally, men taking vasodilators were *more than* four times as likely as other men to be *moderately* impotent.

Although the MMAS found no evidence that anticholesterol (antihyperlipidemic) drugs cause potency problems, this finding is not typical of other investigations. Generally, these drugs are recognized as having a tendency to diminish sexual desire.

Rosenfeld points out that although the law requires that the side efffects of drugs be listed, the rate of impotence reported by the pharmaceutical houses for many drugs is much too low. He believes this is because macho male patients can't bring themselves to tell their doctors, don't know enough to blame the drug, or are afraid of losing the drug if they do report it. Rosenfeld claims that there are at least eighty drugs that physicians frequently prescribe that cause impotence.

Cardiovascular and High Blood Pressure Drugs

Apart from mood-altering drugs, prescription drugs for heart disease and high blood pressure are most likely to have a negative effect on sexual performance. However, their effects are often not easy for doctors to pinpoint. This is because men with high blood pressure often have other health problems (such as atherosclerosis or diabetes) and may have a prolonged background of smoking and heavy drinking.

Diuretics are frequently the first drugs to be tried as therapy for high blood pressure. From 3 to 36 percent of men who take thiazides (hydrochlorothiazide, chlorthalidone, and bendroflumethiazide) have potency problems. Spironolactone at high doses often lowers the sex drive, but less often physiologically affects erections.

Methyldopa (Aldomet) is a synthetic relative of the body's natural precursor of the neurotransmitter dopamine. It's a well-documented cause of erectile problems. Guanethidine and clonidine, which oppose the action of the sympathetic nervous system, also cause problems.

Beta blockers are used for many cardiovascular problems as well as for high blood pressure. In a Medical Research Council study on men with high blood pressure, 13.8 percent more of the men taking propanolol complained of erection problems than those taking a placebo. When a beta blocker causes problems, it should be immediately replaced by a drug of a different class.

Vasodilators help widen arteries and thus increase arterial flow. This would seem to be an erection-friendly activity, and indeed the vasodilator minoxidil (Rogaine) has been so regarded. However, hydralazine, the vasodilator most used for high blood pressure, seems to have a negative effect on erections. But hydralazine is usually used in combination with other drugs, and so it's not clear exactly how these side effects come about.

Calcium antagonists act as vasodilators but, unlike hydralazine, do not need to be combined with a diuretic or beta blocker. It was thought that they might therefore be less likely to cause sexual dysfunction. Although there have been complaints about verapamil, these drugs look promising as a class.

Angiotensin-converting enzyme (ACE) inhibitors (Captopril) make up the only class of drugs for high blood pressure against which there are no complaints about sexual dysfunction. Used over an extended period, they may even improve the arterial supply to the corpora cavernosa and improve a man's capacity to have erections!

Table 1 lists brand-name cardiovascular, high blood pressure, and cholesterol drugs that can cause impotence.

TABLE 1

Brand-name cardiovascular, high-blood-pressure, and cholesterol drugs that can cause impotence

Aldactazide	HydroDiuril
Aldactazine	Hydropres*
Aldactone	Hygroton
Aldoclor	Inderal
Aldomet*	Inderide
Aldoril	Ismelin
Altromid-S	Lanoxicaps
Apesazide	Lanoxin
Catapres*	Lopressor
Combipres*	Metatesin*
Crystodigen	Moduretic
Demi-Regroton*	Norpace
Dibenzyline	Oretic
Diupres*	Raudixin
Diuril	Rauzide
Dyazide	Regitine
Esidrix	Regroton*
Esimil	Salutesin*
Eutonyl	Sandril*
Eutron	Ser-Ap-Es*
Harmonyl	Serpasil*

* Also associated with lowered sexual desire.

Mood-Altering Drugs

Men need to be careful with all mood-altering drugs. Of all drugs, they are the greatest offenders against potency and include uppers, downers, sedatives, stimulants, antianxiety drugs, antidepressants, and sleeping pills. But researchers Alvaro Morales, Jeremy W. P. Heaton, and Michael Condra point out that over time someone has complained about virtually every mood-altering drug, and that it's not always clear whether the drug or the emotional state of the person is most responsible for the sexual problem.

Many mood-altering drugs act on the neurotransmitters and neuropeptides that pass from one nerve ending to receptors on another nerve ending. Thus the drugs may be known by their function as "blockers" or "reuptake inhibitors." This does not mean, however, that they operate with precision only on the neurotransmitters they are meant to act on. To the contrary, their action has been compared to that of a sledgehammer. As well as hitting their target, these drugs unintentionally inactivate a number of other nerve functions, thereby causing what are euphemistically known as side effects. Deep down in the small print of those side effects, you should expect to find the phrase male sexual dysfunction.

Benzodiazepine antianxiety drugs (Valium, Librium) may have male sexual dusfunction as a side effect.

The mood stabilizer lithium can be a troublemaker.

Tricyclic antidepressants are drugs that men should take particular caution with. Imipramine (Tofranil), amitriptyline, and clomipramine (Anafranil) are frequently held responsible for inhibiting both erection and ejaculation.

Monoamine oxidase (MAO) inhibitors such as isocarboxazid, phenelzine (Nardil), and tranylcypromine (Parnate) can also inhibit both erection and ejaculation. Antidepressants of the MAO inhibitor type are notorious for their sexual side effects. MAO inhibitors are prescribed for people with atypical depression—that is, people who feel very depressed but who can cheer up for a while when something good happens. They tend to overeat and oversleep, and while they do not initiate sex, they can enjoy it if their partner makes the first move. After taking an MAO inhibitor for a month, such people begin to feel good and even get their sexual desire back. But after another month of taking the drug, 20–30 percent of both men and women begin to feel side effects.

Major tranquilizers such as fluphenazine (Prolixin), thioridazine (Mellaril), and haloperidol (Haldol) are claimed to inhibit erections in association with a decrease in sexual desire.

The "new" antidepressants—selective serotonin reuptake inhibitors—are thought to behave less like sledgehammers and therefore to have fewer side effects. Serotonin is a neurotransmitter. The best known of the new antidepressants is Prozac, which, in spite of its other benefits, has proved to be the same old story when it comes to negative effects on men's potency. One study found that of the people who received successful antidepressant treatment with Prozac, more than one third developed sexual dysfunction. (But 90 percent of them reported an improvement when they also took the drug yohimbine, which will be discussed in Chapter 9.) According to the *Wall Street Journal*, American pharmacists filled 19 million prescriptions for Prozac in 1995, an 18 percent rise in sales from the year before, for a year's total of $1.47 billion. Presumably, a lot of people taking the drug are men. The makers of Prozac's rival Zoloft acknowledge male sexual dysfunction as a side effect.

Of three even newer "new" antidepressants—Paxil, Effexor, and Serzone—only the makers of Serzone make any claims that it has fewer sexual side effects than its rivals. Two other new antidepressants were expected to win FDA approval later in 1996. In Chapter 11, there is more information on Serzone and on other strategies to use with antidepressants.

Table 2 lists brand-name mood-altering drugs that can cause impotence.

TABLE 2
**Brand-name mood-altering drugs
that can cause impotence**

Anafranil*	Meprospan
Aventyl*	Milpath
Combid	Miltown
Compazine	Nardil
Deprol	Navane
Elavil*	Norpramin*
Endep*	Pamelor*
Eslalith	Parnate
Etrafon*	Permitil
Equagesic	Pertofrane*
Equanil	Prochlor-Iso
Eutonyl	Prolixin
Haldon	Serax
Inapsine	Serentil
Innovar	Sparine
Janimine	Stelazine
Librium*	Surmontil*
Limbitrol*	Taractan
Lithane	Thorazine*
Lithobid	Tofranil*
Lithonate	Tranxene
Lithotabs	Triavil*
Ludiomil*	Tybatran
Marplan	Valium*
Matulane	Valrelease*
Mellaril	Vivactil*
Menrium*	

* Also associated with lowered sexual desire, as are the mood-altering drugs
Adalpin, Asendin, Hanimine, and Sinequan.

Antihistamines

Histamine, a compound produced by the body, makes it easier for substances to pass into and out of the bloodstream. Antihistamines counteract this and help alleviate hay fever and other allergies and common cold symptoms. Antihistamines are also used in many sleeping pills and motion sickness remedies. Table 3 lists brand-name antihistamines that can cause impotence. Table 4 lists other drugs with a similar effect.

TABLE 3
Brand-name antihistamines that can cause impotence

Ambenyl	Mepergan
Antivert	Nico-Vert
Benadryl	Phenergan
Benylin	Remsed
Bonine	Stopayne
Bromanyl	Synalgos
Dramamine	Vistaril
Dytuss	Zipan

TABLE 4
Other brand-name drugs that can cause impotence

Alcoholism drugs	Butabell
Antabuse*	Pro-Banthene
Arthritis drugs	Probocon
Indocin	Regian
	Tagamet*
Bleeding drugs	Uretron
Amicar	Zantac*
Epilepsy drugs	*Glaucoma drugs*
Dilantin	Diamox
Gastrointestinal drugs	*Headache drugs*
Antrocol	Sansert
Arco-Lase	

* Also associated with lowered sexual desire.

TABLE 4 (CONT'D)
Other brand-name drugs that can cause impotence

Infection drugs	Cogentin
Flagyl	Kemadrin
Satric	Pagitane
Muscle spasm drugs	*Prostate drugs*
Flexeril	Estrace*
Norflex	Eulexin*
Norgesic	Lupron*
X-Otag	Proscar
	Zoladex
Parkinson's disease drugs	
Akineton	*Tuberculosis drugs*
Artane	Trecator-SC

* Also associated with lowered sexual desire.

CHECKPOINT

- Some things are so frequently linked with impotence that they can be looked on as impotence risk factors. Some you can avoid, others you have to manage.
- Impotence risk factors can be physical, psychological, or lifestyle—such as having one of the six illnesses named in this chapter, being depressed, or smoking cigarettes.
- Poor health is a greater impotence risk factor than age.
- The six illnesses most often linked to impotence are heart disease, diabetes, high blood pressure, ulcer, arthritis, and allergy.
- It's often hard to tell which is the greater impotence risk factor—the illness or the medication taken for it.
- Check your medication brand names against the danger lists in this chapter.

4

Other Impotence
Risk Factors

We need to keep in mind that impotence risk factors do not condemn us to any particular outcome. By avoiding some and managing others, we can stack the odds in our favor. But in order to avoid or manage them, we must first recognize them for what they are. For example, a heavy cigarette smoker may not easily be convinced that smoking is linked to impotence. He will find it easier to see this as propaganda put out by antismoking zealots. We are often blind to our own faults. May we also be blind to our risk factors? The answer probably is yes, if we enjoy them.

This chapter quickly reviews commonly agreed upon impotence risk factors other than those of the previous chapter. Some of the less well-known risks have longer coverage than the better known. Neither the order nor amount of text indicates any ranking in importance. The most important ones are those that affect you personally.

PHYSICAL RISK FACTORS

Low HDL Level

The total cholesterol level in the bloodstream did not seem to affect potency among the men in the MMAS, but the results for high-density lipoprotein (HDL, or "good" cholesterol) alone were strikingly different. The data implied that men aged 40–55 who suffered from *moderate* impotency could improve their potency to *minimal* impotency by raising their blood HDL level from 30 to 90 mg/dl. Among men 56–70 years old, no one with a HDL level over 90 mg/dl was completely impotent. As the HDL level dropped, the incidence of impotence rose. All the data showed that the HDL level is a strong determinant of impotence.

Smoking

Smoking is used to refer to cigarettes only, and the medical research results given here do not apply to pipes or cigars. This is not a comment on their relative safety, only on what was and was not measured by the researchers.

The MMAS researchers found no correlation between impotence and the number of cigarettes smoked per day, the number of years smoking, or exposure to second-hand smoke in the workplace or home. Smoking in itself did not appear to be a direct cause of impotence, but when smoking was combined with other risk factors, its negative effects were dramatic, as shown below.

- *Men with treated heart disease*. Those who smoked were almost three times more likely to be completely impotent than those who who didn't.
- *Men with treated high blood pressure*. Those who smoked were more than twice as likely to be completely impotent as those who didn't.
- *Men with untreated arthritis*. Those who smoked were

more than twice as likely to be completely impotent as those who didn't.

Since this pattern holds for men taking cardiac and antihypertensive drugs and vasodilators, it can't be said for certain whether smoking was interacting with the medical condition, the medication for it, or both.

The MMAS data also imply that nonsmoking men with treated heart disease who are *moderately* impotent would be *completely* impotent if they smoked.

One experiment involved the effect of smoking on a drug injected into the penis to cause an erection. Papaverine was the drug used; it is discussed in Chapter 13. When papaverine was injected into the corpora cavernosa, it caused blood pressure to build in the spongelike tissue and an erection resulted. Smoking only two cigarettes immediately after the injection was enough to markedly diminish the pressure in the spongelike tissue.

As mentioned earlier, substances in tobacco smoke cause arterial constriction.

Street Drugs

Heroin, morphine, methadone, cocaine, LSD, marijuana, amphetamines, and barbiturates are widely known to affect a man's sexual performance negatively. Street drugs in relatively small quantities may act as aphrodisiacs for some men through their own action or through a placebo effect.

Marijuana appears to seriously interfere with potency in either large single doses or through chronic use. Its psychoactive ingredient, tetrahydrocannabinol, acts on the neurotransmitter dopamine.

One psychiatrist told me that he believes there are more people today with sexual problems than there were back in the 1950s, in spite of present-day widespread sexual information and increased permissiveness. He claimed that drug use is responsible.

Alcohol Abuse

In the MMAS, excessive alcohol consumption resulted in increased minimal impotence. Shakespeare put it more elegantly when he had a character say that alcohol "provokes the desire, but it takes away the performance." After drinking even moderate amounts of alcohol, many men find it difficult to achieve or maintain an erection. Experimental rats given a large dose of ethyl alcohol are almost incapable of having an erection. Drinking a large amount of alcohol at one time may have a direct effect on the powerful neurotransmitter dopamine.

Alcoholism can cause complete impotence. As one of several processes involved in this, alcoholic liver disease profoundly alters hormonal messages between the brain's pituary gland and the genitals. Physicians treating men getting liver transplants have noted that men with nonalcoholic liver disease had normal blood levels of testosterone, follicle stimulating hormone, and luteinizing hormone both before and after the transplant. On the other hand, alcoholic men had various abnormal hormone levels before the operation, which improved after successful liver transplantation.

High estrogen (female) and low testosterone (male) hormone levels are often found in alcoholic men. These men may have breast and nipple enlargement. This hormonal imbalance is probably caused to some extent by liver damage. As the liver ceases to function properly, the estrogen level rises in the bloodstream. At the same time, the liver breaks down testosterone in the bloodstream and inhibits new production by the testicles.

Besides illnesses, the alcoholic is likely to have lifestyle risk factors for both impotence and overall health, such as heavy smoking, abuse of street drugs, poor nutrition, and overeating.

Hormone Levels

Male hormones certainly affect sexual desire and behavior, but their role in the erection mechanism is uncertain. Men with castration levels of testosterone can have erections as potent as men with normal levels.

Of the seventeen hormones measured in the MMAS, only one was found to have a major correlation with impotence. This was dehydroepiandrosterone sulfate (DHEAS), a male hormone made by the adrenal gland. This hormone decreases more rapidly with age than many other male hormones, and is also used to predict cardiovascular disease. No ties to impotence were found in measurements of testosterone or other male hormones, estrogens, prolactin, follicle stimulating hormone, and luteinizing hormone.

The three most frequent endocrinological disorders that may result in impotence are hypo- and hypergonadotropic hypogonadism and hyperprolactinemia, which all involve low levels of testosterone. Men with these disorders respond varyingly to testosterone therapy, which is available in patch form. Two important warnings come with testosterone therapy: (1) older men may have a very slowly developing adenocarcinoma of the prostate, the development of which may be much speeded up with doses of testosterone; and (2) the testosterone therapy may increase a man's sexual desire without enabling him to have an erection, and thereby cause him greater frustration.

Men with hypothyroidism may be impotent; men with hyperthyroidism are more likely to have diminished sexual desire and less likely to be impotent.

Nerve Damage

The more frequent neurologic disorders associated with impotence are spinal cord injury, multiple sclerosis, and peripheral neuropathy due to alcoholism or diabetes. Surgery may interfere with the nerves to the penis and cause impotence. Both prescription and street drugs can cause nerve damage, as can neurological and psychological disorders.

When the upper spinal cord is injured, signals from the brain may not be transmitted to the penis. However, sensory reactions in the genital area may be sufficient to produce an erec-

tion. Therapy with electrical stimulation of nerves is under
investigation.

In order to check yourself for nerve damage, Dr. Steven
Morganstern recommends three self-diagnostic tests to perform at home: the cremasteric reflex test, the ice cube test,
and the BC reflex test. These tests are not conclusive. You need
a doctor's opinion.

1. *Cremasteric reflex test*. This is a test of the neural connections in your pelvic region. You may need assistance to
perform it. Lie naked on your back and stroke a capped pen or
similar harmless object once across the inside of one upper
thigh. There should be a quick upward movement of the testicle on that side of your body. Repeat the test on your other
thigh. Lack of upward testicular movement on either side may
indicate nerve damage in the spinal cord or brain.

2. *Ice cube test*. Place an ice cube against your scrotum for
a few seconds. Your scrotum should contract rapidly. If it does
not, you may have a neurological problem.

3. *BC reflex test*. The BC stands for bulbocavernosus. Insert
a finger in your anus and simultaneously squeeze the tip of
your penis. You should feel a quick contraction of the rectum.
If you do not, your nerves may not be functioning normally.

Overweight

The MMAS found no correlation between obesity and impotence. However, it's generally known that being overweight
is associated with the deposition of fatty deposits on the interior walls of arteries—and that most certainly is linked to
impotence.

Environmental Risks

Heavy metals tend to be toxic when they are ingested or otherwise enter the body. Lead, arsenic, thallium, mercury, anti-
mony, and gold are known to cause impotence.

The following organic compounds are also known to be risk factors.

N-Hexane
Acrylamide
Triorthocresyl phosphate
Methylbutylketone
Carbon disulfide
Dichlorophenoxyacetic acid
Ethylene oxide

Organic solvents in general need to be treated carefully. More controversially, organic chemicals in the environment that resemble some of the natural chemicals in our body have fallen under suspicion. Endocrine-disrupting chemicals, existing in the environment even in minute quantities, if ingested, may mimic natural hormones and disrupt bodily functions. They have been seen as a possible cause of breast and prostate cancers, abnormal fetal development, and low sperm counts. Chemicals that can disrupt the body's hormones and that are widespread on land and in water need to be recognized also as a threat to potency.

The book *Our Stolen Future*, by a scientist, a journalist, and an environmentalist, brought endocrine-disrupting chemicals to the public's attention. Previously, of course, there has been concern about pesticide residues entering the food chain and about the long-term effects of giving domestic animals hormones and antibiotics. The concept of artificial organic chemicals becoming counterfeit hormones and wreaking havoc in our bodies is a striking one. But a number of prominent scientists have come forward to say that that is all it is—a concept. "It's a hypothesis masked as fact," Michael A. Gallo, a professor of toxicology at the Robert Wood Johnson Medical School in Brunswick, New Jersey, told *The New York Times*. Bruce Ames, a professor of biochemistry and molecular biology at the University of California at Berkeley, agreed and added, "It's a political movement and it's based on lousy science." Dr. Ames was a member of a National Academy of Science panel that reported that pesticide residues in food were not important causes of cancer.

Penile Injury

Frank's favorite position was with the woman on top. One night, while he and his wife passionately thrust against each other, their bodies went out of sync and his penis was caught at an awkward angle. He felt intense pain and immediately lost his erection. Next morning, his penis was still painful and looked swollen and discolored. His wife insisted that he see a doctor. In the waiting room at the doctor's office, when the receptionist asked him—opposite all the old people and mothers with young children—why he had come to see the doctor, he was tempted to bolt out the door. If only he knew some medical term for what had happened that would make it sound all right for a respectable 47-year-old accountant. He muttered about a urinary problem and the receptionist gave him forms to fill out. He would never have come if his wife hadn't insisted.

The general practitioner sent Frank to a urologist. When the urologist suggested a minor surgical procedure to relieve the problem, Frank was horrified. "Operate on my penis!" he gasped. The specialist warned him that he needed treatment immediately if he was to avoid future complications. The surgical procedure really was minor, and Frank soon recovered.

Accidents such as Frank's are not restricted to intercourse. Virtually any time a man has an erection, he can injure his penis. He may rupture the fibrous sheath around the corpora cavernosa, rupture a penile vein, or the injury may be less noticeable at first. It happens more often than you might imagine. Irwin Goldstein, a urologist at Boston University Medical Center, told *Men's Fitness* magazine that 3 to 4 million American men may be impotent as a result of penile injury during intercourse.

Dr. Goldstein believes that as many as a hundred thousand American men may be impotent because of penis injuries received from a bicycle seat or crossbar. He points out that half the penis is inside the body and attached to the bone that rests against the bicycle seat. When a man sits on a bike, he puts his entire weight on the artery supplying his penis. When he cycles at 7.5 miles per hour, he is placing a quarter ton of pressure on his penis.

Perhaps the only unusual thing about Frank's story is his prompt seeking of medical care to right the problem. Many men try to ignore the problem and, in time, develop complications, one of which may be Peyronie's disease.

Peyronie's Disease

The first warning may be painful erections. Then a curving or bending of the erect penis develops, which may now also be less hard than previously. Intercourse can become too painful or physically too difficult or impossible to manage.

Perhaps 300,000 American men have a buildup of scar tissue on the fibrous sheath in their penises, a condition known as Peyronie's disease. The buildup of scar tissue causes the erect penis to curve or bend. While the erect penis of most men veers a bit to the left or right, the curvature in this condition is much more radical. In most cases, however, the buildup of scar tissue never becomes so great that the resulting penis curvature interferes with sex.

Surgery to correct the condition is in itself a risk factor for impotence. A procedure called penile plication, which relies on surgical stitches to straighten the penis, involves no risk to potency. Of forty men, aged 17–44, who had penile plication, 96 percent were completely satisfied with the results, according to a study published in the *Journal of Urology*.

Surgery

All of the following surgical procedures have a significant risk of causing the patient later potency problems.

Prostatectomy (for either benign disease or malignancy)
Cystoprostatectomy and urinary diversion
Urethral disruption
Optical internal urethrotomy (but only rarely)
Peyronie's disease
Penile carcinoma
Priapism
Renal transplantation
Colorectal surgery
Vascular surgery
Radiation therapy
Lumbar spinal surgery
Penile amputation
Pediatric urologic procedures

In radical prostatectomies, especially in younger men and in those with less advanced prostate cancer, surgeons can now often spare the cavernosal nerves and greatly reduce the risk of impotence.

Sleep Apnea

People with obstructive sleep apnea, when they are asleep, lose their ability to breathe in air, for up to a minute or more at a time, and then noisily snort in air without waking up. They may repeat this cycle over and over during the night, wakening the next day with a feeling of not having had a good night's sleep. They may feel tired, their ability to learn may be reduced, and their sexual desire may be diminished. In serious cases of obstructive sleep apnea in men, impotence may be a consequence.

Many more men than women suffer from this condition, and most of them don't know they have it. Sleep apnea is associated with snoring and being overweight. Throat and mouth muscles relax with sleep and permit the air passageway to collapse, thus preventing air from being inhaled into the lungs. Oxygen deprivation causes enough bodily arousal to temporarily clear the passageway, but not enough to cause awakening.

Exercising and losing weight are often enough to cure the condition, so long as the person doesn't sleep on his back and doesn't drink alcohol or take sedatives shortly before going to bed. If those measures do not work, professional help should be sought.

Radiation Therapy

Radiation therapy in the pelvic area may be recommended for prostate or bladder cancer. The radiation can cause loss of elasticity in arteries due to scarring, as well as nerve damage. Seed implantation techniques are designed to cause less damage.

Miscellaneous Physical Risk Factors

Priapism, Parkinson's disease, temporal lobe pathology, chronic pain syndrome, and voiding dysfunction can also cause impotence.

PSYCHOLOGICAL OR EMOTIONAL RISK FACTORS

More than 80 percent of all persistent impotence can be traced to one or more *physical* causes, according to Dr. Steven Morganstern. The remaining 20 percent are caused by unknown physical or psychological causes. But even when the cause is wholly psychological or emotional, it is expressed in *physical* terms. That is, some message does not travel along a nerve or some hormone is not secreted into the bloodstream. So long as physical phenomena are involved, medical doctors can be hopeful of finding a remedy.

Much emphasis is placed on the physical today in order to counteract years of people believing that impotence was all in the mind. The Masters and Johnson studies on how sex affects the body are hailed as pioneering work today. Their emphasis on performance anxiety as a cause of impotence, however, strengthened the assumption that impotence was a psychological problem. This led to unpromising scenarios of men searching for psychological problems that they did not have.

Many men occasionally pass through a phase of low interest in sex. No major physical or emotional problem may underlie this state of affairs—although it can become a matter of contention with the man's sexual partner. But if both parties regard this phase as natural downtime, it is likely to pass as unexplainably as it arrived.

It's natural that a man should wonder if his impotence problem has a physical or psychological cause, and there's a simple test that can give him a fairly accurate answer. The test is based on the fact that a healthy man has several erections a night during periods of rapid-eye-movement (REM) sleep. During REM sleep, psychological or emotional problems do not seem to be able to prevent a man from having erections if he is physically capable of having them.

To test himself, a man encircles his flaccid penis with a coil of perforated postage stamps. The stamps should overlap by one stamp and be a comfortable but reasonably tight fit. He moistens the overlapping stamp and uses it to seal the paper ring around his penis. On waking next morning, he can conclude from a paper ring burst open along the perforations that he has had at least one erection and is in physical working order.

Anger

The MMAS found anger to be strongly associated with impotence. The study used the Spielberger scales to measure anger, both suppressed and expressed. Men with maximum levels of anger *suppression* were almost four times as likely as other men to be completely impotent. Those with maximum levels of anger *expression* were almost twice as likely as other men to be completely impotent.

Anger is often associated with disease—for example, peptic ulcer and coronary disease. It may cause heart and vascular problems, arouse nerves excessively, and interfere with smooth muscle relaxation in the penis.

Depression

The MMAS used the Center for Epidemiologic Studies depression scale to measure the condition as major, moderate, or minimal. The study found that 90 percent of men with major depression were either moderately or completely impotent. This compared with 59 percent of men with moderate depression and 25 percent of men with minimal depression.

Depression is often not recognized by the people suffering it and by those around them. This is because the depression may be subtle or its symptoms may be ones not generally thought to be indicative of the condition, such as impotence, loss of appetite, constipation, or inability to sleep. Attempts to cure the symptoms without addressing the underlying problem of depression are not likely to be successful over the long term. On the other hand, once the depression lifts or is treated successfully, the symptoms (including impotence) are likely to disappear "mysteriously." A problem can arise through the use of an antidepressant drug that is in itself a cause of impotence. As we have seen in the section on mood-altering drugs in the last chapter, this cannot be called an unlikely possibility.

There are further complications. Therapists faced with patients who complain of impotence and other symptoms of depression have to consider whether they are impotent because they are depressed or depressed because they are impotent. In real life, it's quite reasonable to assume that a depressed man who develops the symptom of impotence will become more deeply depressed. But even in this case, treating the underlying depression should cause a great easing or disappearance of the symptoms.

Performance anxiety, embarrassment, and constant worry about the problem are some of the "secondary" symptoms likely to appear, as well as depression, in any man who is impotent for whatever reason. When these symptoms are strong, they can take over as the primary cause of impotence, even after the original cause ceases to exist. This mix of physical and emotional symptoms happens to people with a variety of disorders. When something goes wrong in our highly complex systems, it usually causes a few other things to act irregularly also. What is new is the wide recognition given by physicians these days to the links between our physical and emotional states.

No direct link between depression and physical illness has been shown, just as none has been shown for stress. Some physicians see depression not as a direct cause of physical illness, but as making people *vulnerable* to illness. Such complex interconnectedness between multiple factors is only now becoming understood as the basis for bad health—as well as for good health. There is no doubt at all about the strong ties between depression and impotence.

Low Dominance

Dominance is a basic personality characteristic. Men display it in attempting to control their environment and influence others. In the MMAS, men at the maximum level of dominance (measured on a psychological scale) were less likely to suffer from impotence problems. Men with low levels of dominance have low self-esteem and may be expected to interact unsatisfactorily with others in many areas, including sex. This lack of successful interaction may make them vulnerable to impotence.

Experiences and Situations

The MMAS cited anger, depression, and low dominance as the psychological states or emotions most likely to be associated with impotence. Other studies have examined the personal experiences or situations that contribute to men's potency problems. In mentioning these, we need to keep in mind that men often have very different emotional responses to similar circumstances. A thing that arouses anger in one man may cause depression in another man or be met by indifference in a third.

Krane and colleagues regard the following as the most frequent psychological causes of impotence: performance anxiety, relationship conflict, sexual inhibition, conflicts over sexual preference, sexual abuse in childhood, and fear of pregnancy or sexually transmitted diseases.

The NIH panel on impotence adds the following: loss of self-esteem, poor self-image, and increased anxiety or tension with one's sexual partner.

Psychiatric Classification

Psychiatrists use a classification system for mental disorders (they classify impotence without physical cause as one) that they stress is for diagnostic purposes only. The classification system ensures consistency of treatment across cultural and linguistic barriers and in urban clinics where large numbers of people seek help from a limited number of qualified physicians. The classification was put together by the American Psychiatric Association and is known as the *DSM-IV* (for the fourth edition of the *Diagnostic and Statistical Manual of Mental Disorders*).

One psychiatrist warned me that using the *DSM-IV* is a bit like birding with a beautifully illustrated field guide. None of the birds you actually see are exactly like those illustrated in the book. In many years of clinical practice, he said, he had never seen a patient who could be wholly categorized by the *DSM*. He added, however, that the *DSM* gives an excellent academic understanding of how psychiatrists today look at emotional disorders.

The *DSM-IV* divides sexual dysfunctions into sexual desire disorders, sexual arousal disorders, orgasm disorders, sexual pain disorders, and a miscellaneous category. Impotence is termed male erectile disorder and is put in the sexual arousal disorders category, along with female sexual arousal disorder.

Sexual desire disorders consist of hypoactive sexual desire disorder (absence of desire and fantasy) and sexual aversion disorder (aversion to genital contact with a partner). Men with these disorders are capable of erections.

Orgasm disorders are made up of three conditions: inhibited female orgasm, inhibited male orgasm, and premature ejaculation. The two male disorders imply that an erection is achieved.

Sexual pain disorders are composed of dyspareunia (male or female pain during intercourse) and vaginismus.

Male erectile disorder is very distinct in this classification. Again, this classification is solely for diagnostic use, and remedies are not given in the *DSM-IV*. Also, there's no harm in repeating that these disorders are recognized only when no physical explanation—for example, illness or medication—can account for the condition.

CHECKPOINT

- Have your HDL level checked. If it's low, try raising it with diet and exercise.
- Don't smoke.
- Two drinks a day are beneficial to healthy men. If you drink more, dilute them well.
- Some doctors put the physical-psychological cause of impotence ratio at a minimum of 80:20 in favor of physical.
- You can test yourself with a coil of stamps to see if the cause is physical or psychological.
- Anger, depression, and lack of self-esteem are the major emotional problems linked to impotence.

PART II

WHAT YOU CAN DO FOR YOURSELF

5

A More Healthy and Tranquil Life

In these chapters, we look at what we can do ourselves to feel better. We have been looking at individual risk factors—which are not only risks for impotence but for general health. As has been suggested, these risk factors do not operate alone; they interact with one another in both known and unknown ways. If you can neutralize one, you may weaken others. But an array of risk factors can look almost unbeatable, like an opponent's chess pieces in strong strategic positions. In such cases, it's important not to underestimate the innate healing powers possessed by our bodies.

If we give it a chance, our body strives to heal itself. Our body seeks a physiological equilibrium—a state of biochemical balance—in which to function normally. We may be preventing our body from doing that with some of the things we do or the ways in which we do things. If a man has a persistent illness, his body requires medical assistance in the healing process. But even if he's lying in a hospital bed, he's still the one ultimately who must heal himself. By acknowledging this fact, he may become less stressful and more tranquil, more balanced emotionally. While emotional balance does not guarantee physiological balance, it certainly is not at odds with it.

In this aspect of the healing process, a man's spiritual qualities come to the fore. Feistiness and a will to live help many sick people to cope with stress and to awaken previously hidden healing powers inside themselves. Clinical studies have shown this repeatedly.

This chapter is not a survey of mind-body medicine. It is restricted to a few subjects of immediate practical use. As a very brief introduction to alternative medicine, we look at Dr. Andrew Weil's ten principles. After that, we visualize stress as a three-step process that can be managed by mediating any of those steps. Finally, we discuss mindfulness meditation. This is a form of meditation culturally acceptable to men in developed Western countries.

ANDREW WEIL'S TEN PRINCIPLES

Author of the 1995 best-seller *Spontaneous Healing*, Dr. Andrew Weil, has long been a pioneer in expanding the frontiers of medicine. In 1983, he published *Health and Healing* (available in a 1995 paperback edition), which was based on lectures he gave at the College of Medicine of the University of Arizona in Tucson. This book discusses many aspects of wellness and healing that came to change the face of medical expectations in America in the next decade. In one chapter, Dr. Weil mentions his ten guiding principles of health and illness. A quick glance at them gives an interesting and down-to-earth insight into the whole thing.

First, he says, expect to have constant minor ailments in even the best of health. There's no such thing as perfect health, so don't expect it. Second, don't become furious or guilt-stricken when you do get sick—anger and guilt are likely to have neural and hormonal effects that may delay your body's healing. Dr. Weil's third point is that your body heals itself by restoring its lost equilibrium. (There's more on homeostasis or balance in the section on stress in this chapter.)

Fourth, we must be susceptible before a disease agent can

infect us. People resist germs all the time, through their immune system and perhaps by other means we have yet to learn about. His fifth principle holds that there is a mind component in all illness—that is, all sickness is a mind-body phenomenon. Sixth, disease starts small and has its own warning signals. When recognized and treated early, small problems are less likely to grow into big ones.

The seventh principle holds that every body is different. Dr. Weil is not only talking about physical appearances, but also genetic makeup, biochemical individuality, and different susceptibility to illnesses. One consequence of our bodily uniqueness is that there is no such thing as a perfect diet or a perfect treatment. What works for you may not work for me, and vice versa.

Eighth, everyone's body has a weak point. Dr. Weil says his throat is his early-warning system. His throat begins to feel sore when he is low in energy and overstressed, and thus becoming susceptible to illness. Recognizing such personal signals can help us take corrective action and forestall illness before it begins. Ninth, a healthy body needs a healthy blood circulation. All kinds of healing substances travel in the bloodstream, and poor circulation to any particular part of the body is likely to mean trouble. Dr. Weil's tenth principle holds that deep, rhythmic breathing helps balance the body's systems and promotes allover health.

Although Dr. Weil has sometimes been seen as someone at odds with conventional medicine, there's probably nothing in these ten principles that most good physicians would disagree with today. In the early 1980s, however, this was revolutionary talk. And, unfortunately, it remains so for a lot of patients. Nowadays, medically progressive doctors often complain of their medically conservative patients, who, unwilling to change their lifestyles in any way, demand "miracle drugs" to cure what ails them.

The essential message of the new medicine is that people heal themselves. Doctors make possible the opportunity of healing in many cases where it would not otherwise have been likely, but the actual work of recovery must be done by the willing patient.

STRESS AS A THREE-STEP PROCESS

We know from TV, magazines, and newspapers that the stress of modern life is killing us. Experts regularly point out how stress is implicated in many illnesses. People claim that stress made them do various illegal things. Ads promise us ways to escape it. Stress is often made to sound like a killer toxin. The reality is that stress harms some people more than others, and that there's no way to escape stress, only ways to manage it.

The meaning of the word *stress* is fairly ambiguous. When some people say *stress,* they mean something outside themselves that is causing them discomfort. Others take stress to mean the actual discomfort they are feeling. And still others use the word to mean both things. To try to be more precise about what exactly they were saying, many researchers began to use other words to describe what stress consists of. They called an event or stimulus outside a person a *stressor.* The stressor causes the person to feel *distress*. The distress then leads to a *consequence,* which may include illness. Anything that either interferes with or speeds up this stressor-distress-consequence sequence is termed a *mediator*. The diagram shows the process.

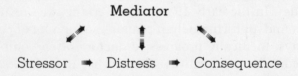

Mediator

Stressor ➡ Distress ➡ Consequence

At first, this might not seem to get us very far. Actually, it provides us with a floor plan of the individual stress problems that we may have. This allows us to manage each problem, instead of trying to ignore it or responding to it with anger.

Seeing stress as a process or mechanism allows us to examine its components more objectively and come up with strategies (mediators) to defuse or alleviate the process. The very fact of having a clearer understanding of what is happening to us is a source of strength to most men.

In using this multistep process, however, we need to keep in mind that we are not little pushbutton cartoon figures who behave according to pattern. A stressor may elicit distress in one person but not in another. The consequence of distress in a healthy man may be a quickened heartbeat, while in a man with coronary heart disease the consequence of similar distress could be anginal pain or even heart failure.

Many bodily and psychological factors influence individual reactions and behavior. For example, a man with a history of high blood pressure is more likely than a healthy man to have consequences involving his cardiovascular system. Similarly, someone prone to anger is more likely than others to respond to a stressful situation with that emotion.

Personality, behavior, social factors, age, gender, ethnic background, and economic status can all be added as mediators to the stressor-distress-consequence sequence. When we make these allowances for ourselves and other people, we can readily understand why we differ in how we are affected by stress, including why some of us stand up to stress better than others.

While doctors traditionally accepted the psychological consequences of stress, the physical consequences (such as illness) are harder to prove because they are more complex and less direct. Only in the last two decades has much attention been given to the links between our brain and bodily systems, including the immune system.

The HPA axis and involuntary nervous systems are the two major communications links between the brain and bodily organs, and thus they are equally major behind-the-scenes players in the drama of male potency. Here we look at how the brain responds to a stressful situation and sends messages to the body by way of these two systems.

HPA Axis

The hypothalamic-pituitary-adrenal (HPA) axis is named for the three hormone-secreting glands that compose it. When the brain perceives a stressor, a signal is sent to the hypothalamus, a part of the brain that acts as a regulator of many bodily functions. In response to stress signals, the hypothalamus secretes cortisol releasing hormone (CRH). Blood within the brain carries the CRH to the pituitary gland, which is often called the brain's master gland because it controls the body's entire hormone (or endocrine) system. The CRH causes the pituitary gland to secrete adrenocorticotropic hormone (ACTH) into the bloodstream. The blood carries the ACTH to the adrenal gland above each kidney and stimulates the adrenal cortex to secrete corticosteroid hormones, such as cortisol.

The hormone cortisol can increase twentyfold in the bloodstream in response to stressors. Cortisol delivers an energy boost by helping to consume fats, carbohydrates, and amino acids as fuels. It also helps release amino acids to repair injured tissue.

Corticosteroid hormones (corticosteroids) regulate cardiovascular functions and have profound effects on all sexual activities. While they help the body react to stressors, they can be a source of problems in themselves if their levels are too high or low. For example, overreaction of ACTH can lead to high blood pressure or diabetes.

A feedback system enables the HPA axis to regulate itself. When the level of corticosteroids in the bloodstream rises above a desirable level, the hypothalamus and pituitary break the cycle of their generation. A failure of this feedback system to regulate the HPA axis can be involved in cases of depression and chronic anxiety.

Involuntary Nervous System

The second major link between our brain and organ systems is the involuntary nervous system. These nerves are of two kinds—sympathetic and parasympathetic—and regulate the parts of our body outside our conscious control, such as our lungs, heart, intestines, bladder, and genitals. The sympathetic and parasympathetic nerves often have opposite effects to each other. For instance, whereas brain messages in sympathetic nerves cause a rapid heartbeat and widening of arteries, messages in parasympathetic nerves result in a slowed heartbeat and a constriction of arteries. (These processes are, of course, intrinsic to the mechanisms of tumescence and detumescence, and the penis is innervated by both sympathetic and parasympathetic nerves.)

The two kinds of involuntary nerves enable the body to function in an automatic and integrated way, in order to maintain a balanced state or homeostasis. The HPA axis and involuntary nervous system are equal partners in adapting and maintaining the body's homeostasis under stressful conditions. The sympathetic and parasympathetic nerves react to stress by preparing the body for fight or flight. The fight-or-flight response, according to the pioneering American physiologist Walter B. Cannon, is a remnant in humans of a stress response mechanism that we share with higher animals. For example, a dog when threatened may stand its ground, bare its teeth, and snarl and be prepared to fight. At any moment, however, the dog may put its tail between its legs and run in flight.

Cannon was the first to describe how both the fight-or-flight response and the maintenance of homeostasis under stress cause the medulla of the adrenal gland to secrete a hormone that is known today as epinephrine or adrenaline. As epinephrine is released, the sympathetic nerves are activated. Together, the hormones and nerves prepare the body muscles for strenuous exertion and for other requirements of either fighting or fleeing. Our rate of breathing increases to supply more oxygen to our bloodstream. Our heartbeat quickens and blood pressure rises, in order to drive blood more quickly to all parts of our body. We lose heat through perspiration, which allows our body to burn more fuel for extra energy. As our blood supply is directed away from our stomach and intestines to other parts of the body where it is more urgently needed, we may feel butterflies in the stomach.

Although these short-term physical changes may make us feel uncomfortable, they enable us physically to meet short-term challenges and are therefore survival aids. In this way, they are normal and healthy. It is only when we are physically responding to a constant barrage of stressors that we risk overloading our involuntary nervous system and possibly running into health problems. But here again, we must remember that what causes distress and health consequences in one person may be only a beneficial stimulant to another. Thus we hear about people thriving on stress.

The death of a spouse is generally regarded as the most traumatic event most people ever have to face. But some physicians claim that we stand up better to major traumatic events than we do to the cumulative effect of minor everyday hassles. The endless small irritations in which modern urban life abounds— such as being stuck in a traffic jam, lateness for an appointment, rudeness of a store clerk, a document forgotten, a key mislaid—build up. After a long day of relatively inconsequential mishaps, a person can be ready to explode emotionally.

There's no way to avoid major loss or traumatic change in our lives, but such events thankfully are infrequent. Most of us can't avoid everyday hassles, either. But there are ways in which we can manage our responses to lessen daily irritants so that they don't build up to volcanic pressure.

MINDFULNESS MEDITATION

There are various kinds of meditation, and some kinds do involve repeating obscure phrases in foreign languages over and over until something happens inside your head. The type of meditation suggested here is another kind altogether. In mindfulness meditation, you step back, for a very short time, from all your activities and try to be conscious of what is happening in your life. Nothing more is involved.

Most of us have much to do and limited time in which to get things done. We tend to perform these tasks mechanically— as if we weren't really there. We simply go about our accustomed ways almost unaware of what we are doing, in a state of forgetfulness or unmindfulness. We may feel at times that things are controlling us, rather than us controlling them. Although this helps us get things done with a minimum of fuss, it also tends to reduce us to feeling like robots or cogs in a machine. We may feel, deep down, that somehow we are cheating ourselves of life.

Jon Kabat-Zinn tackles this problem in his book *Wherever You Go, There You Are*. He recommends stopping whatever you're doing, sitting down, and becoming aware of your breathing once in a while during the day. Perceive what is happening at that moment and ask yourself what you feel. Don't try to change anything, just accept things as they are. When you are ready to move on, be it after seconds or minutes, do so.

It's easy to poke fun at this and thereby dismiss it. It's also easy to overdo it and look foolish. But it's worth trying. Remember the advice to stop and count to ten instead of losing your temper? That has saved some of us from doing very stupid things. And counting to ten is not all that different from listening to yourself breathe. Stopping to take a look at what you are doing and what you really feel about it helps put you back in control of your life. It's a form of power.

Mindfulness meditation also helps you sort out what's valuable to you and what's less so. Some of the insights you gain may be totally unexpected.

Beyond buying you time to calm down a bit, how does meditation help in dealing with a strong emotion like anger? It helps you to become aware of what the anger does to you—how it changes the way you stand and gesture, alters the tone of your voice, and clouds your mind. Kabat-Zinn points out that increasing awareness of anger makes the awareness larger than the anger. The awareness can therefore contain the anger the way a pot holds food.

You no longer vanish into a cloud of rage. You see yourself

being angry. You now have a greater say in the process. If you wish, you have the power to exert control.

CHECKPOINT

- Your body has healing powers of which you may be only faintly aware. But you have to give your body a chance by allowing it to achieve a balance.
- Stress can be a major mind-body health problem.
- Stress can be seen as a three-step sequence:

    stressor ➡ distress ➡ consequence.

    You can interrupt the sequence by mediating any one of the steps.
- The cumulative effect of minor daily hassles may be more stressful than any major event.
- Mindfulness can help you handle daily hassles. Stop now and then and ask yourself what you are doing.

6

Get Fitter

A sedentary lifestyle in itself constitutes a risk factor to health. It needs to be considered as a threat to our well-being in the same way that cigarette smoking and high blood pressure are. If this seems a bit extreme, consider that the Centers for Disease Control (CDC) calculate that a sedentary lifestyle is a contributory factor to about 250,000 death a year in the U.S. A 1991 British Heart Foundation Report implied that lack of exercise needs to be looked at in the same light as smoking a pack of cigarettes a day. The point being made here—since we all know that exercise is good for us—is that leading a sedentary life is living dangerously. If you live like this, count it among your risk factors.

WALK OUT ON A SEDENTARY LIFE

No matter how much of a couch potato a man is, he has to move to some extent—even if it's only as far as the refrigerator. The average person takes about 10,500 steps a day, which totals about four miles. But this does not add up to walking four miles a day! Ten steps here, fifteen steps there—the total builds from morning to night, but we're not talking about arm-swinging striding. In our minimal motions around workplace and dwelling, a lot of us move slowly and deliberately. Some of us barely move enough to keep our joints from seizing up.

For walking to count as healthy exercise, it must be vigorous. Cleaning house can be vigorous work, and it certainly counts as healthy exercise. So, too, is an active home pastime like carpentry. But of all forms of exercise for a sedentary man, walking is the most readily available. All he needs is a pair of comfortable shoes and a little willpower. When it's hot weather, he can walk in the early morning or late evening. When it's cold, he can wear a coat.

If he walks vigorously for twenty minutes four days a week, a man will soon begin to notice a *physical* difference in how he feels. His body is not going to start looking like Arnold Schwarzenegger's, and indeed he probably will not be able to detect any physical improvement when he looks at himself in the mirror, but he will feel better. His body will feel as if it's in better working order. He'll be less stiff getting out of the car seat and less winded after several flights of stairs.

If it's all that easy to stop leading a sedentary life, what's the problem? Why don't more men do it? Most of us enjoy a walk of reasonable length. We can go different places on different days and so not get bored by having to run around the same track every day. We can go alone. We can go with friends. We don't have to get changed into special gear or worry about competing with less than the best equipment. What's stopping us?

Here is the problem: finding the place and the time. Most of us leave home in the morning, work during the day, and return home by car or public transportation. Supposing you can arrange some time for yourself on most days, how about killing two birds with one stone by combining mindfulness meditation and brisk walking? Of course, you may need inactivity to meditate, and you need vigor in walking in order to gain cardiovascular benefit. For many, their requirements may be diametrically opposed. However, mindfulness meditation and walking resemble each other in so far as that they both require you to set aside a time and a place. If you don't, you'll never get around to doing either!

You might try walking part of the way to or from work, by starting out earlier or by getting off at the stop previous to your usual one. For those who peak in the middle of the day, a twenty-minute walk in a city park at luchtime can be very entertaining as well as healthy. A lot of men don't walk in their own neighborhoods because of the wisecracks they would have to endure from acquaintances. But you need never walk so fast that it looks like you are actually exercising, instead of heading purposefully someplace.

There should be no pain—and plenty of gain. You do not need to set plans or schedules for yourself, unless you enjoy having them. Enjoyment is the key word, because if you're not having a pleasurable experience while walking, you probably won't stick with it for very long. Viewing walking as a long-term commitment changes the way you think about it. You're not so upset if you miss some days. You don't develop unrealistic athletic expectations. And, after a while, you get to miss your walks when you are prevented from taking them. Many walkers claim that the first thing they feel when deprived of their daily walk is increased stress. Only when they stopped walking did they realize how effective this mild physical workout was in easing distress from daily hassles.

Feeling fit and healthy, you feel in control of your life. You feel that you have gained in suppleness, strength, and stamina. A loss of suppleness and flexibility is often the first sign of aging in a man's body—or at least is the one most visible to others. When Sam couldn't throw his leg easily over a rail fence or bend down to pick up something without looking as if he might not be able to straighten up again, his friends smiled sadly and recalled livelier days. Sam had just turned 40, and, as it turned out, there was nothing wrong with him whatever except that he stayed home to watch TV these days and rarely ventured anywhere with his friends. Every time they saw him, he looked older and heavier. Happily married with a good job, he devoted his spare time to pro football, hockey, and basketball on TV. The more he watched Brett Favre, Mark Messier, and Michael Jordan physically excel, the flabbier he grew.

It wasn't until Sam lost his job in a corporate downsizing that he awoke from his stupor. Now he made even better money as a consultant, but he had to get out there and compete. Without ever intending it, Sam changed from a sedentary life to a fairly active one solely by walking hurriedly through airport terminals and large car parks several times a week. He and his wife began to see their friends more, and he even let his subscription to cable channels lapse. Sam lost weight and began to look younger, and his friends stopped feeling sorry for him in a hurry.

Suppleness can protect your body from injury, through both agility and flexibility. Strength prepares you for extra effort. As they age, men lose strength. This loss is not as great in a fit body, and with a bit of wisdom in selecting tasks, a man's loss of strength with age can go unnoticed. Stamina keeps a fit man going long after those with unfit bodies have quit from fatigue. Brisk walking for twenty minutes four days a week can supply all three—suppleness, strength, and stamina—with little risk of injury, no boring routines, no equipment like a bicycle, and no special place like a swimming pool. You're fully equipped as you are!

LOOK AT WHAT YOU EAT

Newsweek correspondent Thomas M. DeFrank, at the age of 44, lost forty-seven pounds on the Duke University Diet and Fitness Center program. His blood cholesterol level dropped from 242 to 166. And he amazed himself and his girlfriend with his newfound sexual energy. At Duke, Ronette Kolotkin, Ph.D., studied the sexual effects of weight loss on seventy people, of an average age of 42. She found that a thirty-pound weight loss significantly improved the men's sexual functioning and pleasure. It was, she said, almost as if a renewed interest in sex is the body's way of saying thanks for losing weight.

Most men are aware that the food they eat has a profound effect on their health, and most men are prepared to take *rea-*

sonable measures to achieve a more healthy diet. Their problem is that the experts who write or talk on television about healthy eating seem to live in a different world than they do. Some of these experts count calories—a formidable task for anyone who varies what he has for lunch in a diner or restaurant every workday. Other experts insist on freshness, while every man knows that even when fresh peas are available, the peas he gets while working will always come from a can. The experts have no trouble shopping for all kinds of exotic items and never seem too fatigued to use eighteen ingredients in a dish. Men and their wives do.

Men have a much more common-sense atitude to food than they are generally credited with. They rarely have any use for crash diets to lose weight. Such diets only make the body adjust to famine conditions by slowing down cell metabolism and actually conserving fatty tissues. Any weight lost is soon regained when the diet is abandoned. First of all, men require enough food to create a feeling of satiety. Then they require an instant way to judge food that won't have them poring over a menu like a lawyer over a contract or fiddling with food on their plate like an anorexic.

These two requirements can be met. (1) Eat all the vegetables you want. (2) Three-fourths of your plate should be filled with vegetables, fruits, and grains (complex carbohydrates), and one-fourth with fish, poultry, or lean beef (protein). In a restaurant, ask for extra vegetables and less meat.

Remember, foods that are labeled low-fat may be even higher in calories than the regular versions. A lot of men think that when something is low-fat, they can eat more of it. This applies also to health food and organic food.

Food as Fuel

Human beings are omnivores, as distinct from carnivores or herbivores. Our bodies evolved to eat a variety of foods, and a balanced diet is one with this variety. The various foods provide energy, maintain health, promote growth, and protect us against disease. Most of us eat a sufficiently varied diet and err only on the "provide energy" part. Although most of us have more or less sedentary work, we still eat as though we were turning sod with a plow and a pair of mules from sunup to sundown. We consume food as fuel, don't burn it all up as energy, and store the excess as body fat. Too much body fat promotes clogging of the arteries, diabetes, and other health problems.

The American Heart Association issued some general guidelines on how to structure our daily food intake.

1. Our total intake of fats should be less than 30 percent of daily calories. The average American diet derives about 40 percent of daily calories from fats.
2. Our intake of saturated fats should be less than 10 percent of daily calories. Saturated fats are richer in calories than other foods; we eat less of them and gain more calories.
3. Our intake of carbohydrates should be 50 percent or more of daily calories, and be mostly complex carbohydrates.
4. Protein intake should make up the balance of our daily calories.

Carbohydrates. We use these compounds as fuel for energy. They are of two kinds, simple and compound carbohydrates. Refined sugar is a typical simple carbohydrate, being quickly digested and providing lots of calories and few nutrients. We are unaware of much of the sugar we eat, because it is hidden in soft drinks, cookies, chocolate, and so forth. Complex carbohydrates, on the other hand, are more slowly digested, mostly low in calories, and usually rich in nutrients. Vegetables and whole grains are examples.

Fiber is carbohydrate that is resistant to human digestion. Although fiber has no nutritional value, it makes important contributions to good health. Soluble fiber from vegetables, fruit, and oats helps reduce blood cholesterol levels. By slowing down the entry of glucose into the bloodstream, fiber may be beneficial to diabetics. Insoluble fiber from grain husks and fruit rinds helps our digestive system by binding waste and may protect against some digestive disorders.

Fiber is lost in white flour, white rice, and processed foods. Eat whole wheat bread, brown rice, and fresh vegetables when you can. Drink lots of water, too.

Food Fats. The food fat most likely to cause health and weight problems is saturated fat. Saturated fats are mainly in animal products, including red meat, butter, milk, cheese, and eggs. Cut back on all these as much as you can, for example, by trimming the fat off meat and eating it grilled, never fried. Use canola oil or olive oil.

Protein. Used to build the body's cells, protein is found in meat, fish, and legumes. As adults, our protein needs are relatively small, and the protein we ingest but don't use is stored as body fat.

American Heart Association Diet Guidelines

The AHA has published a set of guidelines to protect your heart. In protecting that organ, you protect most others as well. Here's what the AHA recommends:

- Don't eat more than six ounces of meat, poultry, or fish per day.
- Eat fish or poultry more often than meat, and when you do eat meat, make sure it's lean.
- Cook meatless or low-meat main dishes often.
- Cut back on food fats and vegetable oils, including those in salad dressings and spreads.
- Roast, broil, bake, boil, poach, steam, or microwave food instead of cooking it with fats.
- Eat only three or four egg yolks a week—egg whites are all right to eat in greater quantity.
- Avoid internal organ meats, such as liver and kidneys.

- Eat lots of fruits, vegetables, cereals and grains every day.
- Use skim or 1percent milk and other low-fat dairy products.
- Use salt sparingly.

The Dean Ornish Diet

Dr. Ornish's best-seller *Eat More, Weigh Less* has the even more promising subtitle: *Dr. Dean Ornish's Life Choice Program for Losing Weight Safely While Eating Abundantly*. What more could you ask for? We know there must be a catch. And there is. What you can eat abundantly are complex carbohydrates—that is, vegetables.

But let's look more closely at what he recommends. He significantly uses the term *life choice program* rather then *diet*. This is no fad or crash diet but a consciously chosen change in the way one lives. He points out that our bodies need only 4 to 6 percent of daily calories from fats and believes that the American Heart Association's recommendation of less than 30 percent is much too high. On the Ornish program, you get about 10 percent of daily calories from fats, with almost none of them coming from saturated fats. In fact, he recommends that you become a vegetarian.

He's very persuasive in his reasoning, which describes how calories from fats differ from other calories and how alcohol consumption encourages the laying down of more body fat. All the same, meals begin to sound a bit severe, not to say monastic. This is when the book switches to recipes, many by well-known food writers. These recipes show that you can actually enjoy tasty food without violating the Ornish program.

The Ornish program is probably a must for anyone with atherosclerosis. It could be a lifesaver for the rest of us too, even if we only stay with it for limited periods. One benefit remarked on by a number of men is that, while on it, they lessen their meat habit and taste for fatty foods. When they go back to eating food fried in butter or containing a lot of saturated fats, the food can taste rancid. At this point, awareness sets in that a taste for high-fat food is only a learned taste, not a bodily necessity, as many had previously believed.

The Barry Sears Diet

When overweight men follow the rules of healthy eating and don't lose weight, insulin may be the problem. Barry Sears, Ph.D., approaches this problem in his best-seller *The Zone*. He claims that one in three adult Americans are now obese, in comparison to one in four a decade ago, and that they will not be helped by a diet high in carbohydrates and low in fats and protein. In fact, he says, carbohydrates are a bigger problem than fats for obese people.

The basis of Sears's approach is that our digestive system evolved to deal with protein and fiber-rich vegetables and fruit. Until agriculture developed much later, grains were only a minor part of the human diet. Today, however, grains are the main source of our carbohydrates. A carbohydrate-rich diet causes the body to secrete more insulin, the hormone that reduces the blood sugar level and initiates the storing of unused fuel calories as body fat. This increased rate of insulin secretion can also cause an imbalance among the body's other hormones that regulate physiological functions. The purpose of the Sears diet is to restore hormonal balance.

The word *zone* is used by athletes—and in the book's title—to mean that prime physiological state of the body that delivers the best physical performance. To reach that state, Sears claims we need to eat carbohydrates, protein, and fats in a 4:3:1 ratio. The carbohydrates should be fiber-rich vegetables. We need lots of protein because dietary protein causes the release of the hormone glucagon, which counteracts insulin. We need fats in moderate amounts to slow the absorption of carbohydrates into the bloodstream. The fats should be largely monounsaturated vegetable oils, such as olive oil and canola oil. No more than five hours should pass between meals or snacks, except when sleeping.

Ornish vs. Sears?

Are these two diets in opposition to each other? Is one wrong, and the other right? Is the Ornish diet best for men with cardiovascular risks, and the Sears diet best for those with diabetic risks? These are questions to discuss with your doctor, but don't be surprised if he has no simple answer.

Both these diets have important details not covered in this short look at them. Both are of particular interest to men, because they permit us to eat a reasonable volume of food. If you need to trim down and don't like either of them, you have two other good options: (1) eat less, or (2) exercise more.

ENJOY EXERCISE

Walking breaks the habit of sedentary living and can therefore be a major health-inducing activity. But walking has its limitations when compared to a more strenuous aerobic workout. Various studies have shown that the benefits from strenuous aerobic exercise over time include an increase in sexual desire and frequency of intercourse, greater pleasure from orgasm, fewer sexual problems, and greater self-esteem.

Walking vigorously for two miles every day delivers the increased benefits of more strenuous aerobic exercise. So does swimming for a half-hour three times a week. Because of water's lack of resistance, swimming is particularly recommended for men prone to muscle strains. Your swimming should be rhythmic and relaxed, making use of all your muscles. There's no purpose in swimming timed or competitive laps, unless you enjoy doing so.

Avoiding boredom is an important factor in deciding how you should exercise. Experts advise that the easiest way to

The July 12, 1996, Surgeon General's report on physical activity claimed that burning as little as 150 calories a day in exercise can be an important factor in avoiding serious illness. Here are some of the activities recommended in the report, progressing from less to more rigorous.

- Washing and waxing a car for 45–60 minutes
- Washing floors or windows for 45–60 minutes
- Volleyball for 45 minutes
- Touch football for 30–45 minutes
- Gardening for 30–45 minutes
- Wheelchair propulsion for 30–45 minutes
- Walking 1½ miles in 30 minutes
- Shooting baskets for 30 minutes
- Cycling 3 miles in 30 minutes
- Dancing with a partner for 30 minutes
- Pushing a stroller for 1½ miles in 30 minutes
- Raking leaves for 30 minutes
- Walking 2 miles in 30 minutes
- Water aerobics for 30 minutes
- Swimming laps for 20 minutes
- Wheelchair basketball for 20 minutes
- Basketball for 15–20 minutes
- Cycling 4 miles in 15 minutes
- Running 1½ miles in 15 minutes
- Shoveling snow for 15 minutes
- Stairwalking for 15 minutes

avoid boredom is to choose something you enjoy doing and turn that into your exercise activity. If the physical exertion causes you to pant, it's probably aerobic. Look around, because something new may have come along since you last checked. For example, power yoga has grown in popularity in America in the last few years. This is based on the ancient Ashtanga discipline and consists of moving from posture to posture, without rests, in combinations that give an entire body workout. Almost anyone can do it.

Getting in Shape: Workout Programs for Men & Women, a large-format paperback, has a wide variety of exercises that can be done with a minimum of preparation and equipment, including desk stretches and exercises you can do while on the job or traveling.

By the way, most men burn up about 65 calories for every five minutes of intercourse. But who's counting calories?

Lovemaking Muscles

The main muscles a man uses for thrusting in intercourse are his abdominals (abs). Any small contribution he might make toward them would be for a very good cause. For example, doing crunches strengthens your abs. Lie on your back, with your hands crossed on your chest. Raise your shoulders six to eight inches off the floor, while trying to touch your chest with your chin. You'll feel your abs taking the strain.

A less strenuous way to get your abs moving is simply to tighten and relax them as you lie flat on your back on the floor, with your knees bent and apart.

The PC (for pubococcygeus) muscle contracts reflexively during orgasm, producing many of the pleasurable sensations. Strengthening the PC muscle can amplify these sensations. The PC forms a kind of figure-eight around the base of the penis and the anus. A man uses this muscle to stop the flow of urine midstream. Kegel exercises strengthen the PC. Squeeze the muscle as if you were interrupting the flow of urine and maintain the contraction for about ten seconds. Do this ten times a day. Or you can squeeze your anal region as if you were trying to contain a bowel movement.

QUIT SMOKING

Cigarette smokers know that half of them will die prematurely as a consequence of smoking. According to Dr. Chris Steele in the British medical journal *The Practitioner*, as many as 40 percent of British smokers don't live to collect their pensions, compared with 15 percent of nonsmokers. Government health campaigns, scare tactics, and free clinics have not been enough to motivate all British smokers. But not even life-threatening health problems can do that with many of them. Within six months of surgery, half of all British throat cancer and myocardial infarction patients who were smokers have returned to smoking again.

Experts say that such behavior is typical of addicts, and treatment emphasis is being placed on addiction to nicotine rather than other aspects of smoking. It is not the nicotine itself that harms, but the tars, carbon monoxide, and many of the other 4,700 chemicals in tobacco smoke. It is the nicotine, however, that binds the smoker to his cigarettes, regardless of danger. Milligram for milligram, nicotine is ten times more potent than heroin, according to Dr. Steele. Someone who smokes a pack a day takes two hundred hits of nicotine, which reaches the brain within seven seconds of inhaling and is detectable in all other tissues within fifteen to twenty seconds.

In earlier chapters, we have already seen that smoking is not thought to be a direct cause of impotence, but is linked as a risk factor with a number of other causes. However, from the British statistics quoted above, we have to assume that many men won't quit smoking for the sake of sex! For those willing to try, nicotine patches, gum, or nasal spray, in combination with counseling, seem to have the best results. High motivation of both smoker and counselor is regarded as essential to success.

Dr. Steele says that the three problems of nicotine replacement therapy with patches, gum, or nasal spray are: (1) the person doesn't use them properly; (2) the dose of nicotine given is not strong enough; and (3) the patches, gum, or spray are used for too short a period.

The worst symptoms of withdrawal are felt over the first forty-eight hours, and patches, gum, or spray alleviate these. After that, withdrawal symptoms vary greatly with individuals. Most people speak of bad days and good days, with the good days gradually outnumbering the bad ones.

No doubt those who have stopped smoking have their own surefire tips to offer. Here's mine: I don't believe I could have stopped without having first switched to low-tar cigarettes and cutting down to less than a pack a day. After two years—two years!—on and off the low-tars, I finally quit altogether in disgust. To my surprise, I discovered I had been through most of the quitting already.

CHECKPOINT

- Leading a sedentary life is a risk factor to your general health.
- Break out by walking for twenty minutes on four days a week.
- You need to prearrange a time and place for your walk.
- Eat as many fiber-filled vegetables as you want.
- Find something enjoyable to do that qualifies as an aerobic exercise.
- If you can't quit smoking, switch to low-tars and try again.

7

Aphrodisiacs
and Herbs

APHRODISIACS

A tongue-in-cheek report in the *New York Times* of July 10, 1996, described how young women in the Egyptian city of Mansura, eighty miles up the Nile from Cairo, were transported into sexual frenzy by aphrodisiac-laced chewing gum from Israel. The gum packets carried the word *Spanish* and the drawing of a fly. Some Egyptian newspaper reporters and members of the Egyptian parliament saw in this an attack on the purity of Egyptian youth. Gum seized by the vice squad was tested by health ministry chemists, who could find nothing in it that would lead to sexual arousal.

It's not difficult to understand how a tantalizingly labeled product, allegedly from a traditionally forbidden country, might arouse excitement in women who live in a society in which their individual freedom is held at low value. But does this turn ordinary chewing gum into an aphrodisiac? For those women, in that society, judging by local male opinion, the answer seems to be: Absolutely.

Most men in Western countries, used to the sexual content of advertising and commercial packaging, make a more critical audience. We are slow to believe that something has the power to turn us on sexually—and therefore it doesn't work on us. But are there substances that don't depend on this placebo effect? There certainly are. We will look at some of the natural substances in this chapter, and at drugs in Chapter 9.

Spanish fly (cantharides) is a blistering agent made from ground insects. When taken internally, it has an irritant effect on the genitourinary tract. An irritated bladder, prostate, or urethra can sometimes cause almost continual sexual desire. A safer use of cantharides is in removing warts.

Yohimbe

The FDA classified the West African yohimbe tree (*Pausinystalia johimbe*) as unsafe because the drug yohimbine is derived from its bark. Yohimbine is the only drug for impotence approved by the FDA and is discussed in Chapter 9, along with its possible side effects. Because these side effects can be unpleasant for some men, it is usually better to take the drug yohimbine than the herb yohimbe. The strength of the drug can be accurately measured, while the strength of the active ingredients in the tree bark is more difficult to ascertain.

Potency Wood

Also known as Muira puama (*Ptychopetalum olacoides*), potency wood is a Brazilian shrub that has long been used as a traditional aphrodisiac. According to herb expert Michael T. Murray, potency wood appears to have both physical and psychological impact. At the Institute of Sexology in Paris, France, Dr. Jacques Waynberg conducted a clinical study of 262 men using this herb. Within two weeks, 62 percent of men with a loss of sexual desire claimed improvement, and 51 perecnt of men with erection failures said they had benefited.

GHB

GHB stands for gamma-hydroxybutyrate, a neurotransmitter that heightens tactile sensations all over the body. According to Jordan Freid, who tried out this prosexual drug and others for *Details* magazine, the FDA has restricted access, sale, manufacture, and distribution of GHB, but not its possession. He bought his in powder form by mail order from Italy.

Dosage is tricky. At too high a dose, GHB functions as an anesthetic! Freid had a languid, dreamlike experience, had a long orgasm, and felt intense erotic release.

L-Arginine

The amino acid L-arginine has been credited with harder, more frequent erections, greater staying power, and increased sexual desire. Freid bought his in powder form from a health food store. He took it for four days and noticed only a slight increase in his energy level. A neighbor told Freid, however, that when he took L-arginine, his wife asked him to stop because she became overwhelmed by his amorous advances.

Choline

The B complex vitamin choline helps produce neurotransmitters essential to achieving an erection. Some people are reputed to benefit quickly (increased stamina and greater sexual desire), while others must take it for days or even weeks before they feel a thing. Freid bought his as a citrus-flavored choline cocktail in a health food store. He hadn't expected the cocktail to contain niacin and was unpleasantly surprised by its characteristic short-lived prickly-skin reaction. After several attempts, he abandoned the choline cocktail because of this reaction.

Ginger

The herb ginger (*Zingiber officinalis*), originally from Asia, has been used in the West for two thousand years. Some Chinese herbalists regard it as an aphrodisiac. Herbalists generally regard it as a circulatory stimulant and relaxant of peripheral blood vessels, which would fit in well with an aphrodisiacal role.

Damiana

The herb damiana (*Turnera diffusa*) is used by Chinese herbalists as an aphrodisiac. It can frequently be obtained in the West in Chinese medical remedies, or on its own as a powder or tincture.

Fenugreek

The herb fenugreek (*Trigonella foenum-graecum*) was highly regarded by Hippocrates, and before that is known to have been used in ancient Egypt. In traditional Chinese medicine, it is called *hu lu ba* and is regarded as an aphrodisiac.

Oysters

The claim that fresh oysters on the half shell are a boost to potency is disregarded except by men who swear by them. Oysters have been shown to be rich in the trace mineral zinc, which benefits the prostate gland. (There will be more about zinc in the next chapter.) Before purchasing them, inquire about their geographical origin. To be eaten uncooked, they need to come from unpolluted waters.

Caffeine

In a study of couples more than 60 years old, Dr. Ananias Diokno, a urologist at the University of Michigan, found that those who drank coffee were considerably more sexually active than those who didn't. In the days of harems, Middle Eastern princes used to prime themselves with strong coffee before a visit. Besides coffee, caffeine is found in chocolate, tea, and cola. Casanova ate chocolate to strengthen him in his crowded schedule.

Alcohol and Street Drugs

For most men of average weight, a couple of drinks act as a stimulant. A couple more act as an antistimulant. Knowing when to stop is the trick. With street drugs, the same may be true, except that they are illegal. And an explanation that you were taking the drug for sexual purposes is not likely to gain you leniency in court!

In the 1960s, marijuana earned much of its reputation as a sex drug because people who smoked it were more likely to be sexually permissive. This is not the same thing as saying that it helps in performance. It is also noteworthy that the cheap, low-quality pot widely available in the sixties had a much weaker effect than the later relatively expensive, high-quality product. Many users claim that marijuana enhances lovemaking. Many others claim that the drug causes them to become anxious or withdrawn.

Amyl nitrate, when inhaled, is said to prolong or intensify orgasm, but is not credited with any erection-promoting capability.

Athletes who take anabolic steroids to put on muscle sometimes claim that the drugs make them greater sexual performers. At the University of Pittsburgh School of Medicine, thirty present and past users and fifteen nonusers answered questions on their sexual activities. Those who took or had taken anabolic steroids had intercourse or masturbated more often than nonusers, but they also had more problems in getting erections and maintaining them and in reaching orgasm.

As the street name downers might suggest, narcotics and tranquilizers don't help men achieve erections. Uppers like cocaine and amphetamines can stimulate sexual desire but cause erection problems. The amphetamine derivative Ecstasy is presently popular in the clubs. Taken as pills, it is sometimes mixed with heroin, LSD, or other amphetamines. It is said to give feelings of pleasure and self-confidence and to increase sexual desire. It is also said to give feelings of anxiety and nausea and to cause insomnia and perhaps nerve dam-age. At least twelve deaths have been attributed to Ecstasy.

Herbal Ecstasy

Herbal ecstasy is so named because its effects are supposed to be like those of the amphetamine Ecstasy. The herbal mixture is chemically unrelated to the synthetic amphetamine, and its main ingredient is ephedra. Ephedra has long been used in Chinese medicine for the relief of asthma, hay fever, and chills (the twigs) and for night sweats (the roots). It increases blood flow to the brain, heart, and muscles, and in this it resembles amphetamines. But ephedra is a toxic herb that also interacts with some antidepressants and antihypertensives. Men with heart disease, high blood pressure, diabetes, thyroid problems, or prostate enlargement are warned not to take ephedra. Fif-teen deaths have been associated with herbal ecstasy.

Sexual Sensation

The glans at the head of the penis has the most important role in sexual sensation. The glans transmits the sensations it feels by way of nerves to the spinal cord and then the brain. But the glans is not the only area that can transmit pleasurable sexual sensation in this way. The scrotum, the anus, and the skin around the genital area are all sensitive and linked to the spi-nal cord. Have your loved one give them a try.

Aromatherapy

The vapors of plant essential oils, when inhaled, can stimu-late and relax. You put the recommended number of drops into bath water or massage oil. But go easy on the quantity, because these oils are highly concentrated. If you are allergy-prone, you should test a tiny amount on your skin first. Keep your eyes closed when rinsing or inhaling, and keep these oils out of the reach of children.

According to Angela Smyth, author of *The Complete Home Healer,* aromatherapy with a mixture of these three oils is beneficial for men with potency problems by creating feelings of relaxation and sensuality. Add two drops of each of the following oils to warm bath water or to four teaspoons of massage oil: clary sage, sandalwood, and ylang ylang.

Surroundings

Feeling fit and rested in comfortable surroundings, in the company of a sexually desirable woman, may be all a man really needs—and, for whatever reason, seldom gets. Be active. Active men feel fitter and sleep better. As for the surroundings, go for whatever makes you feel comfortable and relaxed. This is neither the place nor the time to display what a fine family and educational background you have.

Scented candles create atmosphere, although men seem to react less than might be expected to what are regarded as "sensual" odors, such as musk or gardenia. When the Smell and Taste Treatment and Research Foundation in Chicago measured the blood flow to the penises of medical student volunteers, among the aromas that most aroused them (i.e., increased the blood flow) were black licorice, doughnuts, and pumpkin pie!

It must not be forgotten that the greatest aphrodisiac of all is not a substance, but a feeling of love for your partner.

HERBS

Do herbs really work? When someone claims health benefits from the use of a herb or medicinial plant, it's rarely clear whether the benefits really came from the plant remedy or were a placebo effect. So far as the person is concerned, of course, it probably doesn't matter. He got the benefits, regardless of where they came. But would the same plant remedy work for someone who didn't believe in its healing powers?

We don't know the answers to many questions like this about

herbs for several reasons. One reason is that plant biochemistry tends to be extremely complex. Another reason is that we are only now dropping our attitude that plant remedies belong to old wives' tales and folklore.

Cancer prevention is one particular area where plants are known to have beneficial effects. They seem to work as blocking agents in the cancer process. In his book *Healing Essence*, Dr. Mitchell Gaynor has writen about how almost all carcinogens in food remain inert unless triggered by a chemical or special conditions. Blocking agents prevent the carcinogens from becoming activated.

Blocking agents against carcinogens are found in cruciferous vegetables, garlic and other members of the onion family, citrus fruit oils, and caraway seed oil. Many more probably wait to be discovered. The blocking agents work by breaking down precarcinogens and carcinogens into harmless by-products, and by trapping or preventing the formation of free radicals.

Termed phytochemicals, these beneficial plant compounds are being actively investigated by researchers. Tea, particularly green tea, is a rich source of them.

Some phytochemicals act as suppressing agents in the cancer process. Present in cruciferous vegetables, they appear to stop the development of malignant cells, but how they do so is not known.

If plants can successfully prevent the dreaded disease of cancer, it seems reasonable to believe they should be at least as powerful in fighting milder ailments. But it may be many years before we learn which plants are the most effective and why they work. In the meantime, we need to make use of what little knowledge we have and put plants to medicinal use. Physicians often support a patient in his use of plant remedies, as long as these three requirements are met.

1. The plant is nontoxic in the amounts taken.
2. The plant remedy is not substituted for prescribed medications or therapy that the patient finds unpleasant.
3. The plant remedy does not interact with prescribed medications.

The herbs selected here benefit the urinogenital system. The overall good health of this system is, of course, of primary importance to sexual potency. We should keep in mind that since plant biochemistry is complex, not all the benefits of these herbs may be known.

Ginkgo

Extracts from the leaves of the ginkgo or maidenhair tree (*Ginkgo biloba*) have long been a traditional Chinese medicine. Nowadays ginkgo is one of the most widely used herbal remedies in the Western world. Of its many beneficial effects on the human body, the most relevant probably is ginkgo's ability to improve blood flow through peripheral arteries lined with plaque. How ginkgo does this is not known.

R. Sikora and colleagues gave ginkgo to sixty impotent men who had not responded to papaverine injections (to be discussed in chapter 13). Monitoring penile blood flow by duplex sonography, they noticed improvements after six to eight weeks. After six months of ginkgo therapy, the men were evaluated as follows:

50% = Potency regained
20% = Erection now possible with papaverine injection
25% = Improved penile blood flow but still unresponsive to papaverine injection
5% = Condition unchanged

Ginkgo leaf extract is not toxic and has few side effects. This remedy usually must be taken for some weeks before its benefits begin to show.

Ginseng

Korean or Chinese ginseng (*Panax ginseng*) is a small plant widely cultivated in Asia. American, Japanese, and Himalayan ginseng are similar species, but Siberian ginseng is not a member of this family and has different medicinal qualities. The root is used in remedies. White ginseng is dried root, and red ginseng is steamed root. Ginseng and ginseng extracts come in many types and grades. Commercial preparations can be of very low quality and strength.

Ginseng seems to benefit many parts of the body and is widely regarded as a sexual tonic. Research has shown that ginseng promotes testes growth in rabbits and rats, and increases sexual activity in male rats.

Many of ginseng's potency benefits may be indirect. It may help reduce human prostate enlargement. It lowers blood sugar, which is helpful to diabetics. It also helps raise HDL levels. And radiation damage during therapy may be lessened by the presence of the herb in one's system.

Because of varying quality, dosage can be a problem. Ginsenoside is the active ingredient, and its side effects include high blood pressure, anxiety, insomnia, diarrhea, and skin eruptions. But chances are that the ginseng you buy will be too weak rather than too strong. If you live east of the Mississippi and there are woods nearby, you may be able to find the wild American species.

Cranberry

Cranberry juice prevents or helps cure bladder and urinary tract infections, possibly by making the urine acidic. It also seems to help in preventing the formation of kidney stones. Because commercial cranberry juice is loaded with sugar, doctors and herbalists often recommend taking it in pill form. A pleasant-tasting low-calorie version of the juice is now available.

Saw Palmetto

The saw palmetto (*Serenoa repens*) grows along the coast from South Carolina to Florida and in the West Indies. Its berries yield an oily extract that appears to arrest benign prostate enlargement. It is regarded by some herbalists as an aphrodisiac. Saw palmetto extract is not toxic and has no significant side effects.

Pygeum

The powdered bark of pygeum (*Pygeum africanum*), a large African evergreen tree, is traditionally mixed with palm oil or milk. In Western countries, an extract is used. Men suffering from benign prostate enlargement or prostatitis who find discomfort in achieving an erection can benefit from pygeum. This herb can cause gastrointestinal irritation, and this side effect can range from nausea to severe stomach cramps.

Miss Pitman's Tea

For reducing prostate enlargement, Vicki Pitman, author of *Herbal Medicine*, recommends adding a combination of the following to tea: juniper berries, couchgrass, horsetail, and hydrangea root.

Tomato

Dr. Meir Stampfer and colleagues at the Harvard School of Public Health found that tomatoes protect men from prostate cancer. In a six-year study of more than 48,000 men, aged 45 to 75, they found that men who ate ten or more servings of tomatoes a week reduced their risk of prostate cancer by 45 percent. Men who ate four to seven servings a week lowered their risk by 20 percent. A serving is equivalent to a medium-sized tomato or a half cup of sauce. The tomatoes can be raw, juice, sauce, or cooked in food, such as pizza.

This benefit is thought to come from the fact that tomatoes are rich in the antioxidant lycopene, which tends to concentrate in the prostate. Lycopene may combine with free radicals and otherwise discourage carcinogens and precancerous cells.

CHECKPOINT

- Some aphrodisiacs do work, such as yohimbe and potency wood.
- Feeling fit, rested, and relaxed is one kind of powerful aphrodisiac.
- Another is being in love.
- Herbs are great preventives, but ginkgo is certainly worth a try as a potency remedy.
- For preventive plumbing, cook with tomatoes and drink cranberry juice.

8

Vitamins, Minerals, and Foods

The use of vitamins and minerals to supplement the normal diet of healthy people has been a cause of disagreement for three decades now. One side points out that (1) our diet provides more than adequate amounts of vitamins and minerals; (2) evidence is weak that our bodies can benefit from megadoses; and (3) large doses can be toxic.

The other viewpoint holds that (1) the nationally set recommended dietary allowances (RDAs) for vitamins are too low and dietary insufficiencies are widespread; (2) evidence is strong that our bodies can benefit from megadoses; and (3) the amounts that need to be taken, though relatively large, are not toxic.

These differences received initial widespread publicity in the 1960s when Nobel prize winning scientist Linus Pauling advocated large doses of vitamin C as a treatment of the common cold. In mid-1996, vitamin E was the focus of greatest public interest—so much so that stocks were depleted in drugstores and health food stores across the nation. Whatever the validity of the claims for vitamins and minerals, the American public was clearly voting heavily in these substances' favor with its pocketbook.

Even strong supporters are modest in their present-day claims for vitamins and minerals as aids to potency. Some even agree with their opponents, who say there is no scientific evidence that vitamins or minerals directly affect potency. The public, however, disagrees. Anecdotes are widespread about the rejuvenative properties of vitamin E and zinc.

Recall what we said about risk factors: anything that reduces impotence risk factors is a help to potency. By keeping this as our focus of interest, we can avoid the main argument about vitamins and minerals and select items of relevance. For example, evidence exists that vitamins promote peripheral vascular circulation. That would certainly assist potency. Vitamins also seem to help reduce blood levels of LDL (low density lipoprotein—that is, "bad" cholesterol). And the mineral zinc is beneficial to the prostate.

But it needs to be stressed that neither vitamin E nor any other vitamin or mineral seems to work directly as an aphrodisiac—unless, of course, you believe that it does.

VITAMINS

Our bodies use vitamins to build, maintain, and repair cells. Vitamins also help reactions that convert food as fuel into energy. In comparison to nutrients such as carbohydrates, we require only very small amounts of vitamins.

Much of present-day interest in vitamins is in their role as antioxidants. Beta-carotene (a precursor of vitamin A) and vitamins C and E are the important antioxidants. Antioxidants combine with free radicals and thereby neutralize them. Free radicals are atoms or molecules that have lost an electron and that will combine with other substances that offer them one. In doing so, two harmless compounds may unite to form a harmful one. The free radicals originate as by-products of cell reactions, and some are essential to bodily health. Others are suspected to be the chief causes of the physical signs of aging.

Beta-Carotene

Beta-carotene, also known as provitamin A or retinol, is a caro-
tenoid, a relative of the pigment that gives carrots their color.
It is converted to vitamin A in the body. An antioxidant, an
enhancer of the immune system, a cancer preventative, and a
cataract preventative, its chief interest to us is as a preventative of cardiac disease. The research evidence is strong.

In the Nurses' Health Study, organized at Brigham and
Women's Hospital in Boston, 87,000 nurses were asked questions about their food. Those whose diets were richest in beta-
carotene had a 40 percent lower risk of stroke and a 22 percent lower risk of heart attack than those with a diet poor in
beta-carotene. Women who ate five or more servings of carrots per week had a 68 percent lower risk of stroke than those
who ate carrots once per month.

In the Physicians' Health Study, a ten-year study of 20,000
physicians, a subgroup of 333 male physicians with a history
of cardiovascular disease were selected for a beta-carotene investigation. Some took fifty milligrams of beta-carotene every
other day, and the others didn't. Those who took the beta-carotene had half as many heart attacks, strokes, and deaths related to heart disease as those who did not.

In the early 1990s, Dr. Ishwarlal Jialal, of the University of
Texas Southwestern Medical Center, ran a series of laboratory
studies implying that beta-carotene and vitamins C and E
helped reduce blood levels of LDL in the body.

Yellow, orange, and green vegetables and fruits are usually
rich in beta-carotene.

Vitamin C

Vitamin C (ascorbic acid) helps prevent fatty plaque from forming on the interior of artery walls. As already mentioned, it
probably helps lower LDL levels. In high doses, it may help
reduce clumping of blood platelets and their sticking to artery
walls. Vitamin C may also assist in the repair of artery walls,

thereby denying a toehold there for fatty plaque to become attached.

For men with arthritis or threatened by it, vitamin C can help as an anti-inflammatory agent. With inflammation, the body's supply of vitamin C can be quickly used up.

Smokers may gain protection from vitamin C. A laboratory test implied that it protected cells from nitrogen dioxide in cigarette smoke. Men who smoke a pack of cigarettes or more per day may have up to a 40 percent drop in the level of vitamin C in their blood serum and white blood cells.

Many fruits and vegetables are rich in vitamin C.

Vitamin E

Vitamin E (tocopherol), besides its role as an antioxidant, immunity enhancer, and agent against cancer, neurological disorders, cataracts, and arthritis, protects us against cigarette smoke and cardiovascular disease. After all that, would a little help in our sex lives to too much to ask? But despite its reputation as a sex vitamin, there is no medical evidence that vitamin E directly enhances male potency.

Indirectly, however, vitamin E may be extremely important to the mechanics of erections. For example, one of the ways that the vitamin slows down premature aging is by protecting collagen from cross linking. As mentioned earlier, the cross linking of collagen can cause a loss of flexibility in penile erectile tissue walls and in this way contribute to impotence. Slowing this harmful process with vitamin E could make all the difference.

In 1993, findings from the Nurses' Health Study and the Physicians' Health Study were published in the *New England Journal of Medicine*. Through the media, they had a major impact on the public. One finding was that healthy people with the highest intake of vitamin E had a 40 percent lower rate of heart disease than people with the lowest intake of vitamin E. This was thought to be because vitamin E was an agent against LDL. In a World Health Organization survey of sixteen European countries, lack of vitamin E was found to be a higher risk factor for heart disease than either high cholesterol or high blood pressure.

In research on primates, vitamin E was found to act against clogging of arteries. It can break up blood clots. And it may elevate the blood level of HDL. Doing any one of these would make vitamin E a promoter of male potency. Doing them all might restore to it the title of Sex Vitamin, were this not to be misunderstood as Aphrodisiac. To say it once again, vitamin E does not seem to be an aphrodisiac.

Green vegetables, whole grain, wheat germ, nuts, seeds, soybeans, Brussels sprouts, and spinach are rich in vitamin E. Some men switching to a low-fat diet can inadvertantly ingest less than the RDA for vitamin E.

Megadoses vs. Natural Vitamins

Few people would dispute the benefits of beta-carotene and vitamins C and E outlined above, except perhaps to mention that other vitamins are beneficial in other ways. (For example, vitamin A helps produce sex hormones, and vitamin B_6 raises the level of the hormone that regulates testosterone.) Disagreement begins, however, when you wonder how much of a vitamin you need and the best form to take to take in order to gain the benefit. Supporters of high doses of artificial vitamins correctly point out that some of these beneficial effects have only been observed after high intakes of the vitamin. Those who believe in the desirability of vitamins in natural form in our food equally correctly point out that we don't know much about the ways vitamins work in our bodies.

If you decide that you want to take vitamin supplements in high doses, you should discuss it with your doctor. This is so, especially if you have a chronic condition or are taking medication. Vitamins are far more powerful than most herbs, and our bodies are more likely to react to vitamins in unpredictable ways. Vitamins can also interact with other medications.

The Food and Nutrition Board of the National Academy of Sciences, which sets recommended dietary allowances (RDAs) for vitamins, is said to be "reconceptualizing" the criteria by which RDAs are determined.

MINERALS

Minerals are inorganic substances that the body needs in tiny (trace) amounts to assist in various biochemical reactions. The metal zinc is the only one that has been associated with male sexual functioning.

Zinc

A deficiency of the trace metal zinc can result in impaired fertility in men. Zinc exists in high concentrations in the prostate, testes, and semen. A mild zinc deficiency lowers sperm count and motility. A moderate to severe zinc deficiency can lead to shrinking of the testes. A severe deficiency can result in a reduction of sexual desire.

Doctors in Chicago reduced the inflammation of benign prostate enlargement in fourteen out of nineteen men by having them take zinc supplements four times a day. The men showed increases in the zinc concentration of their semen, an indication that the zinc supplements found their way to the men's genitals. Of 200 Chicago men suffering from chronic prostatis not caused by bacteria, 140 responded to therapy with zinc supplements.

Uremic men who became impotent as a result of renal dialysis have had their potency completely restored by taking zinc supplements.

According to Dr. Isadore Rosenfeld, one out of eight American men and women over the age of 55 eats less zinc than the RDA calls for. Because zinc is lost in ejaculation, younger men with very active sex lives should also watch their intake of the mineral.

Lean meat, poultry, fish, oysters, cashews, wheat germ, green beans, lima beans, pumpkin seeds, ground mustard, and nonfat milk are rich in zinc. Dr. Rosenfeld says six medium raw oysters contain 76 milligrams of zinc. The zinc RDA for men is 15 milligrams.

Manganese

According to nutritionist Earl Mindell, the trace metal manganese helps produce two brain neurotransmitters that heighten sexual arousal: dopamine and acetylcholine. Foods rich in manganese include nuts, whole grains, legumes, beets, and green leafy vegetables.

FOODS

Food that resembles either male or female genital organs in shape is likely to have a reputation as an enhancer of sex. Rhinoceros horn and some herbs are thought to be aphrodisiacs because of their phallic shape. But asparagus and celery?

In an article in *Men's Fitness*, Carol Ann Rinzler suggested that you should consider the carbohydrate-protein balance of your meal in view of what you hope will follow. She pointed out that the amino acid tryptophan has a calming effect on the brain. As an amino acid, it is a building block of proteins. In a high-protein meal, tryptophan has a lot of other proteins to compete against in order to reach the brain. The result is that you remain alert—and sexually inclined. But in a high-carbohydrate, low-protein meal, according to Rinzler, tryptophan can float through your bloodstream almost unopposed to reach your brain. The result may be somnolence.

The amount of food you eat may have as much effect on your sexual performance as the kind you eat. John L. Ivy, Ph.D., of the University of Texas, Austin, told Rinzler that when you eat a heavy or high-fat meal, more blood flows to your stomach, where it is needed for digestive processes. This blood may be diverted from other areas, such as the genitals and even the brain, leaving you lethargic and not exactly burning to go the distance.

Octacosanol

Octacosanol, a natural food supplement available in capsule form in health food stores, has a reputation as being a booster of male sexual performance and stamina. It contains wheat, wheat germ, and vegetable oils and is a natural source for vitamin E.

Pharmafoods

In Europe and Japan, pharmafoods—foods that have a pharmaceutical effect, such as lowering cholesterol or blood pressure—are coming on the market. Already, French and Danish yogurts have been reported to lower cholesterol levels, as has a Finnish margarine. Spreading this margarine on toast every morning for a few months is apparantly enough to lower your cholesterol by 10 to 15 percent. At least one medical study backs up these results. It may not be long before pharmafoods have something more direct to offer men in the area of sexual performance. With ultra-conservative FDA policies, however, it may be many years before such products become available on American supermarket shelves.

CHECKPOINT

- You can't get therapeutic quantities of vitamin E from food. You can from an over-the-counter vitamin or, even better, from a multiantioxidant containing beta-carotene, vitamin C and E.

- Eat foods rich in zinc and manganese.

- Try occasional supernutrient special foods. Octacosanol is one with a reputation as a potency food.

9

Drugs

None of these are over-the-counter drugs, and so you cannot take them entirely on your own volition. But you need to be the one who indicates a willingness to try them before many doctors will consider prescribing them. Most doctors will warn you that very little is known for certain about these drugs. There are three major reasons for this: (1) not much research has been done; (2) effects vary widely from individual to individual; and (3) results may be based on less than reliable testimony from participants in tests. In other words, when it comes to being guinea pigs, male humans are less reliable than male guinea pigs.

There is no doubt about the great therapeutic promise of orally taken drugs for potency problems. A pill or capsule can be taken discreetly by a man without his partner's knowledge and therefore without threatening the romantic mood of the occasion, either his or hers. The drawback is that we are only on the threshold. We have not quite yet arrived at this stage.

The FDA has approved only one orally taken drug, yohimbine, for potency problems. Some drugs approved for other purposes have potency benefits and are available. And some drugs under clinical trial can be made available to you, mostly through university hospitals and large medical centers. A urologist can find out where these clinical trials are taking place.

You can go to your local library and look up the same information source about prescription drugs that your doctor uses. This is the annual *Physicians' Desk Reference*, or *PDR* as it is usually referred to. Use the pink pages of the index at the front for generic and brand names. In spite of the technical terms, the descriptions of drugs can make instructive—and occasionally alarming—reading. There are other, more consumer-oriented guidebooks to prescription drugs, but none approach the *PDR* for reliability and comprehensiveness.

The therapeutic benefits of the following drugs are of much current interest.

MUSE

A California company hopes to get FDA approval by early 1997 of a urethral suppository containing synthetic prostaglandin E1 (more about this compound in Chapter 13). The product MUSE consists of a very small applicator that the user inserts into his urethra, at the tip of his penis. He slides the applicator about an inch into the urethra and releases a dissolvable pellet. A man can depend on prostaglandin E1 to achieve an erection, and it has relatively few side effects. This is not a pill, but it's less invasive than an injection.

VIAGRA

At the May 1996 annual meeting of the American Urological Association in Orlando, Florida, clinical trial results were announced for a Pfizer brand-name drug Viagra. The trials were conducted in Britain, and in the largest trial, 351 men with erectile dysfunction were randomly assigned, without their knowledge, to the drug or a placebo. The men on the drug were assigned to particular levels of dosage. The stronger the dose, the greater the benefits reported. Of those on the strongest dose, 88 percent claimed improved performance.

The generic name for the chemical in Viagra is sildenafil. It was being tested to see if it helped relieve anginal chest pain—for which it was not very good—when participants unexpectedly noticed that they were having better erections. In mid-1996, the researchers were getting a worldwide clinical trial under way in which they planned to have 2,500 men who could not achieve an erection take the pill for a year. From their experiences in previous trials, the researchers hope to be able to restore sexual capacity to more than 80 percent of the men.

If all goes well, the drug may become available in Britain and other countries sometime in 1997. With FDA approval, it may become available in the United States in late 1998.

WELLBUTRIN

Wellbutrin is an antidepressant that appears to restore sexual desire. Dr. Theresa Larsen Crenshaw, a specialist in sexual medicine in San Diego, tested the drug in sixty men and women. "It restored dysfunctional men and women to levels of sexual interest we'd call normal," she told *Men's Fitness* magazine. "And a handful had much more dramatic results."

TRAZODONE

The antidepressant trazodone is sold under the brand names of Desyrel and Trazodone. Physicians are warned that this drug can cause priapism—persistent erection of the penis, even without sexual desire. In many cases, surgery was required to correct the priapism, and in some of these cases impaired potency or impotence resulted. Clearly this drug has important properties, but there's a grim irony in the scenario of a man who couldn't get it up becoming a man who can't get it down.

Desyrel has helped a number of men, and is sometimes used in combination with yohimbine. It does not seem to alter the mood of men not suffering from depression.

Other side effects include cardiac arrhythmia. Do not drink alcohol while taking Desyrel.

YOHIMBINE

The drug yohimbine was originally derived from the bark of the yohimbe tree (mentioned in Chapter 7). It is now synthesized artificially and is available in pill form as a prescription drug, the only one approved by the FDA for potency problems. Yohimbine is available under the brand names of Aphrodyne, Yocon, and Yohimex.

According to Dr. Steven Morganstern, yohimbine is thought to increase sexual desire through its influence on the brain and central nervous system. Its help in erections is thought to be due mainly to its role as a blocker of adrenergic neurotransmitters. By blocking these neurotransmitters, yohimbine stops the sympathetic nerves from inhibiting the erection. Yohimbine also promotes an increased flow of arterial blood to the penis.

Yohimbine can increase blood pressure, and it has been known to cause headaches, dizziness, nausea, and anxiety. Nearly all men who take it feel some improvement, and it works *very well* for about one man in every four who try it.

LEVODOPA

A drug for Parkinson's disease, levodopa has also been associated with priapism. It is sold under the brand names Larodopa and Sinemet. In clinical trials, the results have been described as encouraging.

Side effects include involuntary movements, mental changes, convulsions, and nausea.

MINOXIDIL (ROGAINE)

The drug minoxidil was originally sold under the brand name Loniten as a pill for high blood pressure. It relaxes smooth muscle. When people taking it noticed that the drug had the side effect of promoting hair growth, it was tested as a cure for baldness. On getting FDA approval, the baldness remedy went on the market as a solution with the brand name Rogaine. As a solution applied externally on the skin, Rogaine has much fewer side effects than the internally taken Loniten pill.

When applied to the glans or head of the penis, Rogaine and minoxidil solutions have been reported to have beneficial effects on potency. Talk to your doctor before using Rogaine in this way.

Side effects include headache, dizziness, skin rashes, and respiratory and intestinal problems.

TRENTAL

Trental is the brand name of pentoxifylline, a drug for arterial disease that seems to increase the fluidity of blood. In its first clinical trials as an impotence drug, the results were promising.

Side effects include intestinal problems, headache, dizziness, trembling, and chest pain.

NITROGLYCERINE

The simple chemical compound nitric oxide is thought to be an important neurotransmitter inside the penis in the erection mechanical process. Nitric oxide's lack of complexity makes it an attractive target at which to aim therapeutic drugs. A drug that raises nitric oxide levels in the penile erectile tissue (corpora cavernosa) should work wonders.

The explosive nitroglycerine acts in the body as a widener of blood vessels and is used in the treatment of angina pectoris by application of nitroglycerine-containing patches to the chest. Application of these patches to the penis has brought disappointing results. (About half the men found an improvement, but about half also complained of headaches and low blood pressure.) It is thought that the nitroglycerine cannot penetrate the tough fibrous sheath surrounding the corpora cavernosa. (A side problem is that nitroglycerine in the penis can penetrate the vaginal wall and be a cause of headaches. This may necessitate the wearing of a condom.)

Side effects include headaches and dizziness.

MELATONIN

A hormone manufactured naturally by the body, melatonin, when taken as a drug, appears not to have a direct effect on potency. However, its indirect effects may be substantial. According to Doctors Walter Pierpaoli and William Regelson, there is evidence that it interacts with other sex hormones and protects against hypothyroidism. Melatonin also helps prevent benign prostate enlargement and seems to help the body to absorb zinc. Finally, melatonin seems to help in protecting the arteries from being clogged by fatty plaque. Dr. Regelson said that many researchers noted that administration of melatonin caused an increase in sexual desire.

DHEA

A steroid hormone synthesized by the brain, DHEA (for dehydroepiandrosterone) was still mired in mid-1996 by claims and counterclaims for its effectiveness as a drug. In its sulfate form (DHEAS), it was the only hormone level of seventeen measured by the Massachusetts Male Aging Study that had an association with impotence (as mentioned in Chapter 4).

In the September/October 1995 issue of *The Sciences,*
Burkhard Bilger reported an informal remark about DHEA
by Dr. William Regelson, co-author of *The Melatonin Miracle*
and a longtime researcher on both hormones. "The thing that
I've noticed," Regelson said, "is a return of morning erections."
An immunologist sitting across the lunch table nodded and
said, "When I started taking DHEA, the change in my libido
was so striking that my wife and I noticed. It was funny as
hell. I mean, I felt like I was twenty years old again."

OXYTOCIN

Oxytocin is used to induce labor in pregnant women under
the brand names of Pitocin and Syntocinon. Preliminary clinical trials for male potency use are said to be promising.
   Side effects include cardiac arrhythmia and nausea.

NALOXONE

Naloxone (brand name: Narcan) is used to treat depression
caused by heroin or other opiates. Preliminary clinical trials
for treatment of impotence were positive.
   Side effects include sweating, nausea, trembling, and cardiovascular symptoms.

PROPACIL

Propacil (propylthiouracil thyroid inhibitor) is used to treat
hyperthyroidism, which can cause erection problems and loss
of desire. This drug can alleviate the thyroid gland problem
and erection difficulty at the same time.
   Side effects include damage to immune system through
destruction of white blood cells.

What You Can Do For Yourself

PARODEL

Men with a high blood level of the female hormone prolactin
can lower it and enhance their erections by taking Parodel
(brand name for the chemical bromocriptine mesylate). But
they should ask their doctor whether their high prolactin level
is due to a pituitary tumor, which Parodel will not check. Its
usual use is for Parkinson's disease and female infertility.

Side effects include nausea, headache, dizziness, and fatigue.

DOPAMINE PROMOTERS

The neurotransmitter dopamine has long been known to be
important in male sexual performance in animal experiments.
On the other hand, giving male animals dopamine-blocking
substances inhibits their copulatory powers. A number of substances that promote dopamine are also thought to enhance
male sexual performance in humans. Among those currently
under investigation are the following:

Amphetamine
Apomorphine
Deprenyl
Fenfluramine
Methylenedioxy-propyl-noraporphine
Pergolide
Quinelorane

FUTURE OPTIONS

Erection drugs are being tested in skin creams, in patches,
and for use under the tongue, as well as in pills, capsules, and
suppositories. At long last, the commercial viability of conve-
nient products that can deliver is becoming apparent. Terry

Payton, R.N., clinical coordinator of Dr. Irwin Goldstein's urology clinic at Boston University Medical Center, told *Men's Health* magazine, "We'll have an oral pill to help men with erectile dysfunction. There'll be no pain associated with impotence. The only issue will be mustering the courage to see the doctor in the first place."

CHECKPOINT

- Only one drug has FDA approval for potency purposes, but doctors prescribe drugs approved for other uses.

- Most drugs here have been approved for other purposes and are available.

- A drug you can pop in your mouth is a lot more appealing than self-injection or a vacuum device.

- Some of these drugs work better in combination than alone.

- Your biochemistry is unique. Something here may work perfectly for you.

10

Managing Illness as a Risk Factor

Fifty years ago, a man was either healthy or ill, active or an invalid. In those days, doctors could not do all that much for him: "He has a bad heart," people would say. "Don't do anything to upset him." Such a man was fussed over and coddled by those who liked him, and dismissed as being no longer of any account by those who didn't like him.

Although these attitudes have not completely disappeared today, a man with a chronic illness is much more likely to be undetected as such by those who meet him without knowing is background. If this man has found a suitable therapeutic regimen and sticks with it, he can live an active life—working and playing just like everybody else. We take this for granted. Fifty years ago, such statements would have struck most people as naive utopianism.

The difference between then and now is that advances in medicine have permitted us to *manage* our persistent illnesses, some to a greater extent than others. Even though we cannot cure a specific illness and make it go away, never to return, we can frequently hold it in abeyance and enjoy life with just a few precautions.

Again, it comes down to leading an active, nonsedentary life. Keeping both physically and mentally active, within the constraints of good sense, is the key to happiness and good health for everybody.

For each of the six illnesses most associated with impotence by the MMAS—heart disease, treated diabetes, high blood pressure, untreated ulcer, arthritis, and allergy—there are at least several books by nationally known physicians. General agreement exists among medical authorities on the best therapeutic approaches to these six well known disorders. It goes without saying that if you have one of these six persistent conditions, you should be seeing a doctor regularly and be aware of what you need to do to manage your condition successfully.

Dr. Dean Ornish is one of the pioneers of the concepts of reducing risk factors, preventing disease, and managing illness when it does occur. Ornish's message was very powerful—he said it was possible to reverse heart disease and avoid surgery by following a strict very low-fat diet, doing moderate exercise, and meditating daily to reduce stress. In only a few years, he has built a wide following, both among the general public and professional colleagues.

While his program was designed for heart disease, it was immediately obvious that his recommendations for prevention worked equally well against diabetes, high blood pressure, cancer, and many other diseases.

Ornish told the *AARP Bulletin* that, while still a medical student, he noticed how people believed themselves cured after having a bypass or angioplasty. They then went back to smoking, eating animal fat, and never exercising—only to end up in the hospital again in a short time. Ornish knew that heart disease had been reversed in experimental animals and saw no reason why it should not be in humans. Twenty years later, this has come to be the generally accepted view.

"There was a time when doctors paid lip service to risk-factor modification," Dr. Michael J. Horan of the National Heart, Lung, and Blood Institute told the *AARP Bulletin*. "Now it's really being pushed as an important issue."

The strictness of the Ornish diet gets the most publicity, but the program's biggest problem for many people is not that but the daily meditation. Ornish answers complaints about his program's difficulties by saying that it is easier to make big changes in behavior than little incremental ones, because with the big ones you feel better faster. He also feels that the meditation in his program is every bit as important as the diet and exercise.

"The real epidemic in our culture is loneliness, isolation, and alienation," Ornish told the *AARP Bulletin*. "That's especially true for older Americans."

HEARTFELT EMOTIONS

The emotional component in cardiac health is being given the prominence it deserves by a number of clinicians and researchers. For example, James A. Blumenthal, a psychologist at Duke University Medical Center, published a paper in the June 5, 1996, issue of the *Journal of the American Medical Association* on how mental stress tests predicted heart problems better than physical tests, such as the treadmill.

In a study that lasted more than five years, 126 people did mental stress tests that consisted of challenges like solving a mathematical problem in a short time or speaking in public. Of the people who did badly in the mental stress tests, 27 percent suffered a later cardiac event and only 12 percent turned out to be free of heart disease. Regardless of the conclusions of this paper, it is a remarkable demonstration of the mind-body aspects of cardiovascular problems. Diet and exercise alone are probably not enough to reverse heart trouble—a person's way of handling stress must also be altered.

The mindfulness meditation described in Chapter 5 can help you do that.

HEART ATTACKS AND SEX

The chances of a man who has already had a heart attack suffering another one while having sex are about two in a million. So claims a study by Dr. James E. Muller of Harvard Medical School and his colleagues, published in the May 8, 1996, issue of the *Journal of the American Medical Association*.

People with angina or who have had a heart attack previously are no more at cardiac risk during sex than people who have never had heart problems. The study of 858 men and women also showed that engaging in both moderate exercise and sexual activity involved no increase in cardiac risk.

Dr. Robert DeBusk, a cardiologist at the Stanford University School of Medicine, wrote an accompanying editorial on the paper. In it, he defined heart-protective exercise as being equivalent to the exertion required for a middle-aged person to walk up a slight hill, jog very slowly, or cycle at about eleven miles per hour. Such heart-protective exercise, he wrote, could be either done as a single half-hour session or broken up into three ten-minute periods. A fairly fit man's muscles can extract oxygen from blood more efficiently, and therefore his heart has to work less.

Dr. DeBusk stated that the heart rate, blood pressure, and other measures of cardiac stress of active people are lower than those of sedentary people during sexual activity and exercise.

In a *New York Times* report on the study, Jane E. Brody noted that cardiologists have long claimed that sex with one's spouse in familiar surroundings involves no more stress than a short, brisk walk or climbing a flight of stairs. In a study conducted nearly thirty years ago, only 18 of 5,559 coronary deaths were associated with sex, and 14 of those 18 deaths involved extramarital relations. Additionally, nearly all of the 18 deaths occurred after heavy eating or drinking.

HIGH BLOOD PRESSURE:
LIFESTYLE CHANGES

The lifestyle changes recommended for men with high blood pressure would equally help men with heart problems, diabetes, or ulcers. That includes four of the six disorders most often associated with impotence. Here are these recommended lifestyle changes in brief summary.

Lose some weight. Obese men with high blood pressure who lose 5 kilograms of weight can have a reduction in blood pressure of 10/5 mm Hg. This improvement is as good as that credited to drugs in some studies. When weight is lost, not only does blood pressure drop but so do total cholesterol evel, insulin resistance, and cardiac output.

Cut back to no more than two drinks a day. Heavy drinking may be responsible for up to 30 percent of all high blood pressure. Cutting back can bring more or less the same benefits as losing weight.

Reduce your salt consumption by a third. About one and a quarter teaspoons of salt per day would be ideal, according to federal recommendations. Unless you prepare all your own food, this amount would be hard to estimate on a daily basis. This is also the most controversial of the recommended lifestyle changes, with some medical authorities supporting and others opposing a reduction in salt intake. For example, in mid-1996, an article in the prestigious *British Medical Journal* supported American recommendations for a reduced salt intake, while an article in the equally prestigious *Journal of the American Medical Association* opposed it. Incredibly, no basic scientific research has been published on this everyday problem.

Get moderate exercise. This has less measurable effect on blood pressure than it has on cardiovascular health and diabetes. Regular exercise may lower blood pressure. Additionally, the contributions of exercise to the body's overall health must be counted.

Quit smoking. Again, the benefits to cardiovascular health are more striking than those to high blood pressure. While smoking does not seem to affect high blood pressure directly, when a man stops smoking, his blood pressure shows the benefit within months.

Improve your cholesterol levels. Cholesterol levels do not seem to directly affect high blood pressure, either. But getting these levels at healthier values often results in reductions in elevated blood pressure.

As you can see, no simple cause-and-effect deals can be offered. Things are simultaneously complicated and simple. Just take care of your body, and your body will take care of you.

HIGH BLOOD PRESSURE:
TRY AN ACE INHIBITOR

If you have been diagnosed with high blood pressure and often skip taking the diuretic or beta blocker your doctor prescribed because of its effects on your potency, ACE inhibitors may be the thing for you. They don't affect male sexual performance.

Originally isolated from the venom of deadly Brazilian pit vipers, ACE inhibitors—for angiotensin-converting enzyme inhibitors—block angiotensin I from being converted to angiotensin II in the body. Angiotensin I is relatively inactive chemically, but angioensin II elevates blood pressure.

While ACE inhibitors are more expensive and less proven than diuretics and beta blockers, doctors willingly prescribe them because they know that men will keep on taking them. They sell under the brand names of Vasotec, Capoten, and Lotensin. Vasotec and Capoten are also used to treat the related heart conditions of congestive heart failure and left ventricular dysfunction, and Capoten to treat diabetic nephropathy.

Although sexual dysfunction is not a side effect of ACE inhibitors, they have some others. The two most frequently heard complaints are: (1) on taking the first dose, you may have a

sudden drop in blood pressure and feel dizzy; and (2) about
one in twenty people taking ACE inhibitors develop a dry
cough. ACE inhibitors can also interact with other medications and with alcohol.

But these are minor complaints. Where it matters—in the
bedroom—ACE inhibitors know their place.

ARTHRITIS: NONDRUG THERAPY

When you begin to suffer significant side effects from drugs,
talk to your doctor about them. All you may need is a change
of dosage. If that doesn't help, your doctor can prescribe another drug. The fact that he gave you a drug with unpleasant
side effects doesn't mean your doctor doesn't know what he is
doing. He's possibly giving another patient a higher dose of
the same drug with no evidence of side effects. It's a matter of
individual biochemistry.

Having a persistent condition often makes the taking of
medication almost inevitable, especially if the condition is
painful, as in arthritis. Besides finding the right medication
and the minimal effective dosage for your individual case, you
can keep an eye out for nondrug therapy that might ease your
reliance on medication.

Massage is one such therapy being investigated for the alle-
viation of arthritis. Prof. Tiffany Field, of the University of
Miami School of Medicine and head of the Touch Research
Institute, has found evidence that massage lowers the blood
levels of some stress hormones and increases those of pleasure hormones, including mood-enhancing endorphins.

In one study conducted by Prof. Field, children with rheu-
matoid arthritis were massaged daily for a month. At the end
of that time, they had lower blood levels of the stress hormone
cortisol than previously, and suffered from less pain and stiff-
ness. In mid-1996, she was planning a clinical study on adults
with osteoarthritis in hope of similar results.

"One of our main goals is to see if we can decrease the need for painkillers," she told R_x *Remedy* magazine. "Massage is not a substitute for standard medical care but it may turn out to be an important supplement."

STOPPING ALLERGIES BEFORE THEY START

Researchers are developing new vaccines to stop allergic reactions before they can get under way. Available vaccines—immunotherapy shots—make use of extracts of ragweed, pet dander, and other natural allergens. These vaccines are not wholly effective, need to be repeated, and can sometimes cause dangerous reactions themselves.

As reported by Marilyn Chase in the *Wall Street Journal*, Dr. Philip Norman of Johns Hopkins University is experimenting with vaccines that use protein fragments instead of natural allergens. Two of these vaccines—against cats and ragweed—are being tested by ImmuLogic Pharmaceutical Corp. of Waltham, Massachusetts.

Other vaccines under trial aim at the master switch of allergic reactions—immunoglobulin E (IgE). Switch off IgE and there is no allergic reaction. Tanox Biosystems Inc. of Houston is testing a vaccine against hay fever, and Genentech, Inc., of South San Francisco is testing one against bronchial asthma. Many biotechnology companies, research institutes, and medical centers are testing others.

CHECKPOINT

* Managing stress is every bit as important as diet and exercise.
* Someone who has had a heart attack is no more likely to die while having sex than anyone else.

- There's no increased cardiac risk in following moderate exercise with sexual activity.

- Cheating on their partners after heavy eating or drinking is what kills men during sex!

- ACE inhibitors lower high blood pressure without interfering with your potency.

- Nondrug therapy can reduce your dependency on medication.

- Look out for an opportunity to join a clinical trial of a new allergic reaction prevention drug.

11

Reducing Other Impotence Risk Factors

Although we tend to talk about risk factors as if they were independent entities separate from one another, this is not how they operate in real life. Risk factors are related and interdependent. Emotional risk factors may be tied to physical ones. These relationships may be obvious or difficult to detect, and unique to an individual or very common. Beyond this, the following study reveals how positive and negative factors can be linked—and how we can make use of our strengths to protect ourselves from our weaknesses.

MODERATELY FIT SMOKERS VS. SEDENTARY NONSMOKERS

Smokers who had high blood pressure and high cholesterol but were moderately fit lived longer than nonsmokers who were healthy but sedentary. This result was drawn from an ongoing longitudinal study of 25,341 men and 7,080 women by Dr. Steven N. Blair and his coworkers. Dr. Blair is director of research for the Cooper Institute for Aerobic Research in Dallas. The participants were studied over periods that averaged eight and a half years. The study appeared in a July 1996 issue of the *Journal of the American Medical Association.*

"It's the first study to show that low fitness is at the top with smoking," Dr. Blair told the *New York Times.* "It's a more powerful risk factor than high blood pressure, high cholesterol, obesity and family history."

Both low fitness and smoking nearly doubled the risk of early death for men and women, Dr. Blair went on. While lack of fitness is not usually considered as a risk factor for impotence, perhaps it constitutes a very important indirect one. As we have seen earlier, some level of moderate fitness can be very helpful in regaining male vitality.

The study also found that moderately fit nonsmokers had a 41 percent lower mortality rate than sedentary nonsmokers.

Moderately fit people get some exercise nearly every day, Dr. Blair said, for example, by walking 1½ miles in 35 minutes, bicycling 3 miles in 30 minutes, or gardening for 30 to 45 minutes. If you yourself smoke or care for someone who does, these might be numbers to keep in mind.

STEVE SOBEL'S
FIVE WAYS TO MANAGE STRESS

Steve Sobel, Ph.D., author and founder of the New England Institute of Stress Management, contributed these five pointers to an April 1996 issue of the journal *Advance for Medical Laboratory Professionals.*

1. Commit yourself to peaceful coexistence with all the idiocy and idiots around you in your workplace.
2. Never lend your car to someone who is your offspring.

3. Tame quails mindfully. That is, enjoy life in the here and now. Tomorrow will arrive, even if you don't worry about it.
4. "If you can't sing good, sing loud!" (He's quoting Forrest Gump.)
5. Drink cranberry juice, which he says helps your level of optimism as well as your urinary tract.

I feel better already.

MANAGING ANGER

The Massachusetts Male Aging Study found that anger was the greatest emotional or psychological risk factor for impotence. This included both anger expressed and suppressed. Managing (rather than controlling) anger is a complex matter, because not all anger is bad. Indeed, justified anger has been the stimulus for some of men's greatest actions. Anger that inspires you to protect an old woman from a mugger is admirable. Leaning on the horn every time a car cuts in front of you in city traffic is not.

Clearly, the occasional rescue of an old lady is more a risk factor for a man's life than his potency. In fact, since a successful rescue would boost his self-esteem, occasional anger may contribute to potency. But the constant use and reuse of hormones and nerves in frequent bursts of irritation at minor stressors seems to do the opposite.

One widely held belief is that it is better to let off steam than to hold it in. This is possibly true, but the only real solution is not to build up steam in the first place. Referring to expressions of anger like flipping a middle finger, Duke University psychiatrist and author Dr. Redford Williams told *Men's Fitness*, "The more you engage in these kinds of venting behavior, the more likely you are to get angrier the next time. It increases your aggression."

He suggested that before joining in a confrontation with

someone, people should say how much they value or respect their opponent. Then they should describe the transgression, explain their feelings, and underscore the consequences. Next they have to give the other person a chance to speak. Then a compromise may be possible.

Gilda Carle, Ph.D., runs corporate workshops on anger. She told *Men's Fitness* that it's important to step back and try to view the anger-causing incident more dispassionately. This gives you a chance to figure out if it's really the incident or something else that's responsible for your anger. Stepping back also gives you a chance to differentiate between foolish confrontations and worthwhile ones.

Dr. Williams said that hostile personalities never completely get rid of their anger. "It's always there, particularly when you get tired," he said. He himself still has an occasional lapse.

ANGER: MORITA AND NAIKAN THERAPIES

Psychotherapist and author David K. Reynolds, Ph.D., has tried to incorporate some Eastern viewpoints and therapies into our Western lifestyle. He calls this approach Constructive Living. He points out that Western therapists try to make their patients feel good about themselves, so that they can then make positive changes in their lives. The Eastern attitude, on the other hand, is that you make positive changes in your life first and then you feel good.

In his view, we make a mistake by trying to "fix" a negative emotion such as anger. This does not work because our feelings are uncontrollable, and we end up confused and frustrated. Instead of trying to change our feelings, he believes we should just accept them and go on as adults with our responsibilities.

For facing anger, he makes use of two Japanese psychotherapeutic techniques, one active—Morita therapy, and the other reflective—Naikan therapy. Morita therapy was developed by psychiatrist Morita Shoma in the early 1900s.

Yoshimoto Ishin, a businessman who became a temple priest, developed Naikan therapy in the 1930s.

Morita therapy. This could be called keeping busy. Here is how it works with anger: The next time you become angry with someone, instead of shouting or simmering, paint a wall or wash your car. When your anger subsides, you will have something to show for it.

When you develop feelings of stress because of all the things you have to do immediately, make a list of them and then calmly proceed to do them in alphabetical or any other order you prefer. Don't look at the list and wring your hands. Just start at the top and work your way down.

Enjoy doing things for themselves and don't back away from something new. In fact, on certain days, deliberately go out and do something you have never done before.

Naikan therapy. According to Reynolds, this reflective approach to anger balances the active approach. It involves spending twenty minutes or so at the end of the day thinking over the good things that have happened to you, remembering kind things that people did for you and you for them, and also recalling any hurt that you caused others. (Angry individuals may have a bit of trouble with this initially.)

If someone you see often causes you to become angry frequently, be polite and respectful at every meeting with him or her. Do small favors for people you like, especially things they won't know you did. Try to see the positive things people do all the time and how much you have to be grateful for. You can only see these things by looking outside yourself.

Regardless of how effective they are in moderating his anger, trying to put these two therapies into effect should give a man some interesting insights into himself. That in itself may provide him with greater control in unforeseen ways.

Another interesting thing about the Morita and Naikan therapies is that they require a man to commit himself to doing something about his anger. That may be the biggest step of all.

MANAGING THE SIDE EFFECTS
OF MEDICATION

When a medication is effective for a man's ailment but, as a side effect, it causes him potency problems, he has at least six options. These options, as they related to antidepressants, were discussed at the May 1996 annual meeting of the American Psychiatric Association and reported in the *New York Times* by Jane E. Brody. The six options are as follows. Obviously, these options must be discussed with a doctor for each individual case.

1. *Lower the dosage*. A possible drawback here is that the medication may lose or have diminished effectiveness.

2. *Engage in sex just before taking daily dose*. At this time, the drug is at its lowest strength in the body, and presumably its side effects are also reduced. Having sex by the clock, though, upsets many people and may require skill in explaining to newly met partners.

3. *Take yohimbine or another potency drug*. This can work well, although no drug available now is completely consistent and dependable.

4. *Take medication in combination with drug to combat its antipotency side effects*. This biochemical balancing act is not all that easily achieved.

5. *Take weekend holidays from drugs*. Take the last dose of the week on Thursday morning and resume at noon on Sunday. This may not be advisable to do with all medications.

6. *Change medications*.

Dr. Anthony J. Rothschild, a psychiatrist at the Harvard Medical School and McLean Hospital in Belmont, Massachusetts, tested the fifth option—weekend holidays from drugs—on thirty patients who took a serotonin-reuptake inhibitor antidepressant and suffered side effects of sexual dysfunction.

He told the meeting that patients taking Zoloft and Paxil showed a significant improvement in sexual function during the drug-free period, but that patients on Prozac did not, because that drug takes too long to wash out of the body. Their brief abstinence from drugs did not cause any worsening of their depression.

Two reports at the meeting dealt with the option of changing medications—both from the antidepressant Zoloft to Serzone. In one study, the change caused a robust improvement in sexual desire and improvements also in other aspects of sexual function. In the other study, patients who stayed on Zoloft were found to be more than twice as likely to experience sexual problems than patients who changed to Serzone.

UP WITH THE BIRDS

Men who suffer from stress, fatigue, and distractions may be at their sexual best when they wake after a night's rest, with high blood levels of male hormones. Indeed, switching from night to morning lovemaking may be the only tonic required.

CHECKPOINT

- Even if you can't quit smoking, moderate exercise may save you after all.
- Maybe you should be less solemn about stress.
- Don't lose your temper—instead, try the Morita and Naikan therapies.
- You have six options in handling unwanted side effects from medications.
- First thing on waking, try having sex.

PART III

WHAT YOU CAN DO WITH WITH PROFESSIONAL HELP

12

Seeking Professional Help

YOUR REGULAR DOCTOR

If you get yourself in reasonable physical and emotional shape and there's still no sign of you regaining sexual vitalty, it's definitely time to seek professional help. Even if you have seen signs of improvement, a doctor's suggestions for further progress may be invaluable.

Before seeing a doctor, you may need to consider confidentiality. This is almost never a concern with the doctor himself or his staff. But if he is a school or company doctor, his paper and computer patient files may be accessible to others without his knowledge.

If you are a member of a HMO, you may be required to see your primary health provider first. Be candid with him. He will examine you before recommending that you see a urologist. In some cases, he may be able to solve your problem without sending you to a specialist. Going to any general practitioner or family doctor will be the same as going to a HMO doctor. Their expertise lies in general diagnosis and in screening for other medical problems of which you might not be aware. When a regular doctor sends you to a specialist, it will be understood by the specialist that he has performed this initial screening of you. So be cooperative and forthcoming. Your regular doctor will probably not be an expert in male potency problems, but he may spot something that an expert might miss. He might also decide that you need to see another specialist—for example, a cardiologist—before seeing a urologist.

When you see a regular doctor and explain your problem candidly to him, as a competent physician he should respond to you in the following ways.

- He should take your sexual problem as seriously as he would a lung or kidney problem. But don't be offended if he tries some humor. He may be trying to put you at ease or even covering up his own shyness on sexual matters. If he is dismissive of your problem or tells you it is not a medical matter, you need to see another doctor. If he tells you that impotence is part of the aging process, run for the door.

- He should show a keen interest in any illnesses you may have or previously have had, particularly in any symptoms of cardiovascular problems, diabetes, and high blood pressure.

- He should question you about your use of medications, street drugs, and alcohol.

If your doctor proceeds along these lines, you need to place your trust in him, volunteer any information that might be helpful, and take whatever tests he deems necessary. He will almost certainly not be able to offer any diagnosis or recommendations until the results of your blood tests come back from the lab.

If your regular doctor says that you do not need to see a urologist, he should be able to make you understand why and provide the remedy himself. If he is a HMO doctor, he may be under pressure not to make referrals to specialists. Doctors in group practice are sometimes slow to send patients to specialists outside their group. If you are sent to another doctor within the group, know what his specialty is and why you are seeing him instead of a urologist. If you do not understand the reasons why, insist on seeing an outside urologist.

Lastly, when your regular doctor arranges for you to see a specialist, inquire what kind of specialist you are seeing and why. If you live near a major medical center, you have a better chance of being referred to a urologist with a subspecialty in male potency problems.

SEEING A UROLOGIST

If you have no regular doctor and your medical insurance terms do not require you to see one first, you can see a urologist from the outset. You will find how to contact one in the "Where to Get Help" section at the end of this book. A urologist is both a surgeon and physician, trained specially in disorders of the urinogenital system. The subspecialty of male potency problems is relatively new, and some urologists are much more aware of recent developments than others.

A urologist may ask you to bring your spouse or sexual partner with you on your first visit. This is simply to get an understanding of your problems from another viewpoint. Many men make poor describers of their situations. You will have to fill out a long medical questionnaire. Your interview with the urologist will go into intimate detail on your physical sex life, your beliefs and emotions, your home and job situations, how you handle stress, and so forth. A reader of this book will see the purpose of many of the questions. The more forthright and truthful you are, the more the urologist can help you. And don't think you could tell him something he hasn't heard before!

Some urologists are easier to talk to and confide in than others. But this is a comfort you may have to do without. Tell him everything. Don't wait to have the intimate details dragged from you. If it helped, you'd make sure a judge heard all the evidence, even if he lacked charm. Make sure the urologist does, too.

The urologist will give you a physical examination, particularly of the genitals. Then samples of your blood, urine, and prostate fluid will be taken for lab tests. As with the regular doctor, you cannot expect to hear much until the lab results come in. In addition to regular lab tests, you should undergo a screening for diabetes and a hormone screening (testosterone, luteinizing hormone, follicle stimulating hormone, prolactin, and possibly sex hormone binding globulin). You can also expect to undergo some of the urological tests described below.

On your second visit, the urologist will discuss the test results with you, name the probable causes of your problem, and recommend a course of action. If more tests need to be done, a third visit may be necessary. In recommending a course of action, the doctor should suggest the least invasive and dangerous procedures first. You—and your spouse—need to be well informed about all your therapeutic options, including their effectiveness, possible complications, and costs.

You can use this book as a reference to what therapies you have already tried yourself and what you are most interested in trying now. Ask the urologist which drugs in pill or capsule form he has found most successful in his practice. If a pill or capsule works for you, you do not need to take an injection.

Injection of Vasoactive Drug

In this test, the doctor injects a vasoactive drug into the penis (more about this in the next chapter). An erection should result. If one does not, this could mean that arterial blood to the penis is being blocked or that the mechanism for closing off veins from the penis is not working and that venous leakage is taking place.

Dynamic Infusion Cavernosometry

You wil recall that the corpora cavernosa are the paired cylinders of erectile tissue in the penis. The doctor injects a vasoactive drug into the corpora cavernosa to cause an erection. He measures the amount of continuing drug infusion needed to maintain the erection or, using saline to maintain pressure, the time it takes for the erection to be lost after the infusion is stopped. From these measurements, he can draw conclusions about the arterial supply or venous drainage. This test usually indicates that the doctor is considering surgery.

Cavernosography

Cavernosography works on the same principle as arteriography. The doctor injects fluid into the corpora cavernosa and follows its circulation on x-ray films. This technique is effective in detecting venous leakage and in seeing how the hardened lumps of Peyronie's disease affect the erectile tissue.

Arteriography

This test is performed when the doctor suspects that arteries to or in the penis are clogged or blocked and that surgery may be necessary. A harmless liquid is injected into the arterial system and x-rays are taken of its distribution pattern in the genital area. Blockage sites show clearly on the x-ray film, and the amount of blockage is visually evident.

BC Reflex Test

This unforgettable test was one of three self-diagnostic tests for nerve damage described in Chapter 4. It involves inserting a finger in your anus and simultaneously squeezing the tip of your penis. The correct response, signifying intact nerves, is a quick contraction of the rectum.

Nerve Conduction Tests

In these tests, the doctor uses electrodes to detect electrical impulses in the penis, pelvis, and spinal column nerves due to the BC reflex. Uncharacteristic or absent impulses would suggest that something is wrong in the nerves that carry messages back and forth between the penis and brain. These tests resemble the checking of circuits in electrical or electronic devices.

Biothesiometry

This test measures the sensitivity of the penis skin. Having placed a small instrument against the penis skin, the doctor gradually increases its vibrations until the patient can feel them. The doctor notes the level of vibrations and repeats the test several times on other parts of the penis. From this he can tell how well the nerves that carry skin sensations are working. These nerves may be damaged most often in diabetics and alcoholics. This is not a test of the nerves connecting the penis to the spinal cord.

Duplex Ultrasound with Pulsed Doppler and Color Flow Sonography

Simply by pointing a device at the penis, the doctor can use ultrasound and the Doppler effect to measure blood flow in the penile arteries and veins. Measurements may be taken before and after injection of a vasoactive drug into the penis to cause an erection.

Snap-Gauge Band

The Snap-Gauge band tells whether a man has nocturnal erections. A normal, healthy man has three to five erections a night, each lasting twenty-five to thirty-five minutes and usually occurring during periods of rapid-eye-movement sleep. The Snap-Gauge band consists of a ring containing three plastic filaments that is placed around the penis before going to sleep. It works like the self-administered test with a coil of postage stamps, in that nocturnal erections break a constricting ring. With the

Snap-Gauge band, the rigidity of the penis can be measured by the number of plastic filaments broken.

When filaments are broken, it can be assumed that an erection is physically possible and that emotional or psychological causes prevent erections in waking hours. In some cases, however, even when an erection is physically possible, vascular problems may still be responsible for potency difficulties.

The Snap-Gauge band, because of its low cost and convenience, has widely replaced the older, more elaborate equipment needed for nocturnal penile tumescence monitoring. The Rigiscan device is also widely in use.

PSYCHIATRIC SELF-ASSESSMENT

When most people first go to a psychiatrist, they think the big question is whether they are normal or crazy. They find it hard to believe that this is not what is foremost on the psychiatrist's mind, since it is on theirs. But *normal* and *crazy* are social judgments, not psychiatric ones.

If you visit a psychiatrist with an erection problem, his questions are likely to be along the following lines. By answering these questions, you can play at being your own psychiatrist:

Is your erection problem real?
  Do you have unreasonable sexual expectations for a man your age?
    Do you think your erections should be as frequent now as when you were 20?
    Do you think you should be able to have a full erection at will?
  Are you sure you are not suffering from premature ejaculation?

Is your erection problem the symptom of another problem?
  Do you suffer from major depression?
  Do you abuse alcohol or street drugs?

Do you have any other sexual disorder?

Do you have low sexual desire?

Do you feel aversion to the sexual act?

Are psychosocial factors contributing to your erection problem?

Were you under stress just before you failed to get an erection?

Do you live at constant high levels of stress?

Are you going through a period of marital discord?

Is your spouse emotionally and physically available to you?

Are psychosexual factors contributing to your erection problem?

Are you sexually attracted to your spouse?

Have you any interest in same-sex relationships?

In lovemaking, do you and your spouse have different preferences, such as position or at night or morning?

Do you suffer from performance anxiety?

Is it possible that your spouse is sabotaging your lovemaking?

Do you think your spouse has any sexual problems?

Do you regard yourself as sexually well informed?

Are you knowledgeable about the mechanics of sex?

Did you get adequate penile stimulation?

Did too much penile stimulation cause premature ejaculation?

PSYCHOSEXUAL THERAPIES

Behavioral sex therapy has largely replaced traditional talk therapy for cases of psychological or emotional impotence. Modern therapy aims more at correcting the immediate causes of impotence rather than the deep underlying psychological causes. But whatever therapy is used, the male emotions most often associated with impotence remain the same. Most psychiatrists and psychologists agree that they are as follows. You could even call them emotional risk factors for impotence.

Anger
Depression
Anxiety
Fear
Apathy or boredom
Disgust or repulsion

A sex therapist usually depends on behavioral conditioning or some method related to it, while a sex counselor usually relies on more traditional one-on-one or group sessions. But sexual psychotherapy is not regulated in the way many other therapeutic fields are, and you have to be leery of con men, prostitutes, and crackpots. One good way is to have your urologist recommend a therapist or counselor to you, but make sure that he has sent patients to this person before and achieved satisfactory results. Another way is to see a sex therapist or counselor affiliated with a good hospital near you.

Psychiatry

Many people confuse psychoanalysis and psychiatry. The modern psychiatrist may or may not be a psychoanalyst. Many are not, and their ideas have advanced well beyond those of Freud. The two years of talk sessions before real problems emerge belong to psychoanalysis.

The methods of a psychiatrist are difficult to summarize because he is always a qualified medical doctor and thus has a wider access to knowledge and methods, including writing prescriptions, than any other kind of practitioner. The "Psychiatric Self-Assessment" in this chapter and the section on "Psychiatric Classification" in Chapter 4 provide an introduction to the psychiatric approach.

A psychologist with a Ph.D. is not a medical doctor and cannot write prescriptions. However, he may have received much more intensive training in a particular field than an M.D. The problem is that someone can receive a Ph.D. in almost anything, and you have no way of knowing if your therapist got his in computer science or botany! Many therapists have no academic qualifications.

Cognitive Behavioral Therapy

Therapists in this field see sexual activity as a set of behaviors that can be changed by direct behavioral intervention and learning (cognition). Individualized treatment is more effective than a programmed approach, and the man's spouse or sexual partner is usually encouraged to participate. In fact, couples therapy is often regarded as the most effective. Behavioral training today would probably consist of some combination of the following.

Basic sex education
Skills training
Cognitive restructuring
Relaxation training
Assertiveness training
Individual therapy
Couples therapy
Communications training
Structured home practice assignments

Systemic Intervention

When other forms of therapy fail for no apparent reason, a therapist who uses systems theory may provide the solution. Many of the approaches are the same as or similar to those of cognitive behavioral therapy. One important difference exists— the therapist looks at the couple as a system. As a system, they have the potential of developing circular forms of negative behavior that can neutralize just about any therapeutic intervention. Unless the therapist sees the couple as a system, he may not observe what they are doing to each other.

Desensitization

This is a form of conditioning or behavioral therapy in which the man is asked to view a series of images that he finds stressful to look at. The images become stronger or more explicit as they are shown to him. As he gets used to them, the images cause him progressively less stress. Even more powerful images may follow after he has been "densensitized" to the previous ones, and the process is repeated. One desensitization study of men with potency problems claimed some improvement in 75 percent of the participants.

Biofeedback

Biofeedback for erection problems involves the electronic monitoring of a man's penis, so that he can see for himself on a video screen the effects that erotic images have on him. Use of the system in various ways may help him to achieve erections. Although it has been shown to be beneficial to men with high blood pressure, biofeedback is still at the experimental stage in erectile problems.

Hypnotism

Two different approaches have been used with apparently promising results. In one approach, attempts are made to give the man under hypnosis an erection. In the other approach, hypnosis is used to reveal some deeply repressed experience or emotion that may be causing the impotence.

Sensate Focus Therapy

The fundamental purpose of this therapy is to create a sense of trust and safety between the couple, to lessen the fear of failure, and to change the emphasis from performance to plea-sure. To achieve these goals, the couple is asked to give up all attempts at intercourse for the time being. This allows the man to concentrate on intimacy and sensory pleasure rather than on performance.

This approach is used today in different ways and to differ-ent extents by various therapists. Sensate focus therapy devel-oped from the pioneering Masters and Johnson studies of the 1960s. In the Masters and Johnson version, the treatement lasted for fourteen consecutive days and the participants were urged to treat it as a vacation!

One of the appealing aspects of this form of therapy is that it places the man in a win-win situation, because if he does not attempt intercourse he is following the therapist's instruc-tions, while if he does have intercourse he has scored a suc-cess! But what if he tries and fails? The therapist can explain that he tried too soon.

Surrogate Sex Partner

A partner is needed for sensate focus therapy, but many men with impotence problems no longer have a partner. Masters and Johnson attracted media attention back in the 1960s when they provided them. To this day, prostitutes use surrogate sex therapy as a cover, whereas the real health professionals in this field get scarcer because of fear of AIDS. But because of their amazingly high success rate, surrogate sex partners re-main an important option for the partnerless man. Ted McIlvenna, Ph.D., president of the Institute for Advanced Study of Human Sexuality in San Francisco, attributes a 90 percent success rate to surrogates.

Joe Kita wrote an excellent article on surrogates, called "Sub-stitute Teachers," for the May 1996 issue of *Men's Health*. Ac-cording to Kita, a surrogate charges about $100 per hour for weekly two-hour sessions. Initially, she and a new client talk over the phone, after she has received information on him from the therapist and he has cleared his AIDS test. If they get along conversationally, she makes an appointment for them to meet, usually at a cozy apartment she keeps for this purpose.

After some small talk, they go to the bedroom and undress. They lie naked on their backs in the bed, holding hands. She leads him through a series of relaxation exercises, allowing the man's stress to lessen. A surrogate told Kita that, in her opinion, most male problems are based on men's stereotyped bedroom notions and inability to relax with a woman.

When she feels that the man has relaxed, she softly massages and explores his body with her fingers. She tries to engage him in communicating to her what he likes sensually. The first visit ends not in passionate intercourse, but in a direct exchange of intimate communications. Both report independently to the therapist. The second visit starts out like the first but ends up going as far as the man wants to take it. On the third visit, the surrogate and her client go over what he has learned so far. After that, the number of visits depend on the needs and progress of the man.

CHECKPOINT

- Your medical insurance policy may require you to see a regular doctor before seeing a urologist.
- If your doctor doesn't take you seriously, take a walk.
- Don't be put off seeing a urologist to save your insurance company money.
- Use what you read in this book to talk with your urologist. Insist on discussing all your options. If he dismisses some, understand why.
- Are you normal or are you crazy? In psychosexual therapy, chances are you'll never get to lie on a couch and recall your unhappy childhood.
- Call them anything you like, but don't call surrogates unsuccessful.

13

Caverject

According to Dr. Cameron Lockie, the idea of giving men an erection by injecting drugs into the penis originated in an accident. In 1978, someone dropped a syringe loaded with the drug papaverine, and the projectile fell needle first into a male patient's penis, delivering a charge of the drug into it. He got an erection. And a new era dawned . . .

Clinical studies of the effect of vasoactive drugs (drugs that affect blood vessels—in this case, drugs that cause erectile tissue to dilate) injected into the penis got under way in the early 1980s. Some drugs worked better than others, but the process worked. Now, for the first time, a method was available by which the majority of men could rely on having an erection at a particular time.

VASOACTIVE DRUGS

Research continued through the 1980s into the 1990s, and is ongoing today. Among the drugs used in this research, the following have been prominent.

Papaverine. This is an alkaloid from the opium poppy, but is not an opiate and not habit-forming. It relaxes the smooth muscle of vascular walls. It may also stimulate the action of the neurotransmitter VIP in the penis.

Phentolamine. This compound interrupts the passage of a neurotransmitter (it's an alpha-adrenoreceptor antagonist) and causes smooth muscle to relax. For convenience, such compounds are often called alpha-antagonists.

Prostaglandin E1 and E2. These compounds act in ways similar to hormones and are direct smooth muscle relaxants. They are available in both natural and synthetic forms. As substances produced naturally by the body, they appear to have fewer side effects than other vasoactive drugs.

Atropine. This compound interferes with the neurotransmitter acetylcholine and relaxes smooth muscle.

Phenoxybenzamine. An alpha-antagonist.

Trazodone. An antidepressant that acts as an alpha-antagonist. This drug was previously mentioned in Chapter 9.

VIP. This amino acid residue is metabolized by the body. Some researchers think that it is a key neurotransmitter in penile erection.

CGRP. Another amino acid residue metabolized by the body, it is a potent vasodilator.

Linsidomine. A vasodilator.

These drugs were used singly and in combination with others. For example, Dr. Fred E. Govier and his colleagues, at the department of urology of the Virginia Mason Medical Center in Seattle, published a study of successful triple-drug therapy in 1993. They used a combination of papaverine, phentolamine, and prostaglandin E1. Doctors Glenn S. Gerber and Laurence A. Levine, of the University of Chicago, had published a landmark study in 1991 using prostaglandin E1 alone. Finally, after years of research and clinical studies, the natural form of prostaglandin E—alprostadil—received FDA approval in July 1995 to be marketed by prescription as an intracavernous injection drug for erectile dysfunction. It is sold under the brand name of Caverject.

SOME PROS AND CONS
OF SELF-INJECTION THERAPY

Upside

- In a 5- to 7-year follow-up study of men self-injecting vasoactive drugs published in 1992, J. C. K. Chan and colleagues could find no directly related harmful side effects.
Most men were very satisfied with the therapy. They had
no systemic complications and not much pain from injections or erections. Their main complication consisted
of intracavernosal (inside the corpora cavernosa) masses
that were related to the number of injections but that did
not interfere with sexual satisfaction.

- Dr. Christine Evans, a urologist at Glan Clwyd Hospital in Rhyl, Wales, in September 1995, had some patients who had been injecting themselves with successful results for up to eleven years without any problems.

- For men who do not have a steady partner, self-injection therapy is easier to conceal than use of a vacuum
device and ring (see next chapter).

- Self-inection works regardless of whether impotence
has physical or psychological causes.

Downside

- Pain is felt from the needle and physical damage is
caused to the penis by frequent injections. But with
Caverject, both pain and damage are minimal.

- Most people find their partner's arousal during foreplay arousing to themselves and also affirming. A
woman who sees that her man's arousal is chemically
induced may be sexually turned off because she feels
she is not the source of his arousal.

- Although little or no evidence exists that intracavernous
self-injection causes emotional or psychological prob-

lems, an interesting possibility has been mentioned. A healthily functioning man has to feel sexual desire in order to have an erection. A man using intracavernosal self-injections can have an erection any time, even when he doesn't feel like having sex. If he injects out of duty rather than desire—and if this becomes a regular pattern—the possibility exists that his sexual desire will decline and he will begin to avoid sex. Again, this was mentioned as a possibility, and not something that has been observed.

PRIAPISM

Dr. Dudley Seth Danoff, author and urologic surgeon at Cedars Sinai Medical Center and UCLA School of Medicine, claims that, in his practice, self-injection has restored thousands of "penis-weakened" men to an active, fulfilling sex life. He tells of one extremely wealthy man in his sixties who had a reputation as a lover and had recently married a beautiful woman twenty years younger than himself. A vascular condition caused him to become impotent. Dr. Danoff taught him to self-inject papaverine. Things went well, and the man spent time away at his home in Europe and on his yacht in the Mediterranean. When he came back to Los Angeles, he told Dr. Danoff that he was having the best sex he had had in thirty-five years—three times a day, sometimes for hours at a time.

Dr. Danoff became concerned. He had instructed the man to inject himself no more than once every other day. This was the sort of misuse of the therapy that could result in priapism. Priapism is a rare condition but a threatening one. Blood trapped under pressure for too long in the penis can irreparably damage the erectile tissue and result in impotence beyond the remedy of vasoactive drugs.

Dr. Danoff asks patients to phone immediately if their injection-induced erection lasts longer than two hours. An injection of Neo-Synephrine into the penis causes gradual detumescence. He often gives patients a syringe preloaded with an emergency dose.

CAVERJECT

A paper called "Efficacy and Safety of Intracavernosal Alprostadil in Men with Erectile Dysfunction" was published in the April 4, 1996, issue of the *New England Journal of Medicine*. Despite its somewhat daunting title, it got widespread media attention. The paper was written by Otto I. Linet, M.D., Ph.D., Francis G. Ogrinc, Ph.D., and a nationwide group of collaborating physicians. They claimed that the therapy sold under the brand name of Caverject was effective and had tolerable side effects. Here at last was a safe, dependable, unobtrusive way for an impotent man to have an erection. The media had good reason to be interested.

The paper was based on three separate studies: a dose-response study, a dose-finding study, and a study of efficacy and safety. Each was conducted at multiple sites and involved impotent men ranging in age from 20 to 79. The diagnosed causes of impotence in each study are shown in the table:

Diagnosed causes of impotence

Cause*	Dose-Response Study	Dose-Finding Study	Safety Study
Vascular	44%	36%	57%
Neurological	13%	24%	13%
Psychological	14%	16%	10%
Mixed	29%	23%	20%

* Both vascular and neurological causes may originate with diabetes.

In the six-month efficacy and safety study of 683 men, 86 percent of the men were satisfied with the therapy. The amount of time of each man's erection depended on the dose he received. Doses could be set to give an erection for about an hour.

Penile pain was the main side effect. In the dose-response study, 23 percent of the men reported pain; 69 percent, in the dose-finding study; and 50 percent, in the efficacy and safety study. The pain in most cases was mild, and only a few men dropped out of the studies because of it. As a prostaglandin, alprostadil is thought to be pain-sensitizing. Although the drop-out rate in these studies was very low, it is thought to be much higher among ordinary users of Caverject. Perhaps half stop injecting it within a year.

In these studies, a single case of priapism occurred and was successfuly treated. Among other side effects, 5 percent of the men had prolonged erections, 2 percent had penile fibrotic complications, and 8 percent had hematoma or ecchymosis.

Referring to Caverject, Dr. Perry Nadig, a urologist in San Antonio, Texas, told the *Wall Street Journal*, "It's an easy technique . . . with relatively little pain."

But pain may not be the issue. "It just isn't something that provides much romantic fantasy appeal," said Dr. Abraham Morgentaler, director of the male infertility and impotence program at Beth Israel Hospital in Boston. "Everyone would love a pill to treat impotence problems."

A pill it is not. In the next section, we will look at what exactly is involved in Caverject therapy.

Self-Injection Procedure

The prescription drug Caverject comes in two strengths and is sold in six packs of injection kits. Each injection kit is con-tained in a blue plastic box about the size of an eyeglass case and may be stored at room temperature for up to three months. The kit consists of vial of Caverject powder, two alcohol swabs, and a syringe with a needle attached and prefilled with steril-ized water.

Having wiped the rubber stopper of the powder vial with an alcohol swab, you inject the syringe water into the vial. Without removing the needle, you gently swirl the vial until all the powder is dissolved in the water.

Keeping the needle tip below the fluid level, you draw the fluid back into the syringe. Get rid of air bubbles and pull the syringe out of the vial.

The paired corpora cavernosa extend along each side of the penis shaft from below the bulbous head nearly to where the penis meets the body. They are cylinders containing erectile tissue. The drug relaxes the smooth muscle lining the spaces in the spongy erectile tissue, and this allows arterial blood to rush in, pressure to build, and an erection to form.

You inject on one side of the penis only, alternating the side and varying the site with each injection. Sitting, hold your penis by its head and stretch it lengthwise along one thing so that you can see the injection site. Swab the site and push the syringe needle in until the metal part is almost entirely inside the penis. Slowly push down on the plunger. When the injection is complete, pull out the needle and apply pressure on the injection site with the alcohol swab until bleeding stops, usually after three to five minutes.

You can safely dispose of the syringe and vial by replacing them in the blue plastic case and using the red locking device. They cannot be recycled.

Within minutes, you will feel an erection begin to grow.

Combinations of vasoactive drugs continue to be of major therapeutic interest. One frequently used combination is alprostadil, papaverine, and phentolamine in varying proportions, sometimes called Tri-mix.

There are tricks to learn and skills to develop in the technique of self-injection. For example, allowing the alcohol on the penis skin to dry completely before injecting removes much of the pain. Using the smallest gauge needles you can find, such as ones used for insulin injections, makes a big difference in damage caused to tissues. You have to watch out for veins in the penis skin, because breaking one with the needle can leave the skin looking bruised and discolored for days.

Self-injection may not be the most romantic prelude to love, but it's an enabling act. As Dr. Irwin Goldstein of the Boston University Medical Center told *Men's Health* magazine, "Any treatment—even if it involves needles, even if it involves surgery—beats no sex at all."

CHECKPOINT

- You have to inject Caverject, but it's by far the most reliable therapy to achieve an erection presently available.

- Being able to depend on Caverject more than makes up for its mild discomfort and inconvenience.

- Self-injection is not hard to conceal from a new partner.

14

Vacuum Constriction Device

Kevin was a 22-year-old student, vegetarian, and disbeliever in modern medicine. He was seeing a doctor because he was impotent and had no other choice. He refused to supply any medical history, other than to say he was in good health, and refused to submit to any tests other than a physical examination. The doctor gained no information on why he was impotent or for how long.

"I want no drugs," he told the doctor. "I won't let you put anything in my body."

The elderly doctor was amused by the young man's truculence and felt sorry for him in his plight. The doctor also remembered an unsolicited medical video he had received in the mail a few weeks previously and not yet viewed. After a physical examination, which turned up nothing unusual, the doctor suggested that they watch the video together. It showed how to achieve an erection through the use of a vacuum device. Kevin was skeptical and said it was probably an actor in the video who had no real-life problem. But he agreed to go to have a trial demonstration with a specialist.

158

A few months later in the doctor's office, on a day with a very heavy schedule, Kevin showed up unannounced and said he had to see the doctor. The doctor agreed to see him between appointments. Kevin walked into the doctor's private office with a stunningly beautiful girl in her early twenties.

After shaking the doctor's hand, Kevin said, "I want you to meet Alice."

The doctor shook her hand, Kevin gave him a big smile, and the young couple left. For a moment, the doctor wondered why Kevin hadn't just phoned instead. Then he saw that Kevin, in his own highly personal style, had found a more imaginative way of saying, Thanks, Doc, I'm feeling better.

HOW IT WORKS

The vacuum constriction device (VCD) consists of a cylindrical vacuum chamber, which looks like a length of transparent plastic pipe, open at one end for the insertion of the penis. The closed end of the vacuum chamber is attached to an electrical or hand pump to create the vacuum.

The penis is covered with a water-soluble lubricant, particularly at its base, where an airtight seal must be established. After the penis is inserted into the vacuum chamber, the pump is turned on. The vacuum causes the penis to become rigid after a few minutes. The best results are obtained by running the pump for a minute or two, turning it off for a very short spell, and running it again for another three or four minutes.

Withdrawing the penis from the chamber breaks the vacuum. To maintain organ rigidity, an elastic ring or rubber band is worn around the base of the penis. The ring or band can be kept around the open end of the vacuum chamber and slipped down around the penis before it is removed.

An erection by this method can be maintained safely for about thirty minutes. Then the elastic ring or rubber band should be removed to avoid risk of damage to erectile tissue within the penis.

USER SATISFACTION

Dr. Christine Evans finds that rings and vacuum devices have improved over the last few years, but are still "fiddly." According to her, they are successful in 70 percent of cases. Other physicians report 80 to 95 percent satisfaction rates. One study demonstrated higher penile blood pressure after six months' use of the VCD, and there are reports of spontaneous erections in men who have been using the VCD for six months to a year.

Most men are happy with the erections they get from a VCD. Rigidity, frequency of intercourse, and partner satisfaction have not been faulted by the majority. As a result, many have higher self-esteem and a sense of well-being.

Some men feel discomfort on ejaculation, and others remark on penis numbness or coldness or on difficulties in ejaculating.

The VCD works for men with an implanted prosthesis that is no longer functioning. The VCD can also be used in combination with intracavernous injections.

Physicians often suggest that a man's spouse or partner should be in on the decision to purchase and use a VCD. As with intracavernous self-injections, partners may feel left out and unstimulated sexually themselves. If a couple can make the VCD part of their foreplay, this will do much to restore spontaneity to their sexual activity.

Like Kevin's doctor, physicians generally suggest that a man has a personal fitting of a VCD by a specialist, rather than rely on the package instructions or a video.

VCD VS. SELF-INJECTION

- Both VCD and self-injection work regardless of whether the cause of impotence is physical or psychological.
- Men have reasonable cause to fear that a woman will

be put off if she learns that the man she has just met
uses self-injection or a VCD. Most men would feel more
assured breaking the news after having made love successfully at least once. Self-injection has the advantage
of being much more easily concealed than a VCD.

- Both the VCD and self-injection have a very high drop-
out rate among users. This seems to have less to do
with the techniques themselves than with a lack of romance and spontaneity in using them. This is probably an area in which a man should rely on a woman's
empathy and imaginative suggestions.

- Making your therapy part of your love life is far easier
and safer to do with a VCD than with self-injection. No
injuries with a VCD have been recorded.

- In a twelve-month study that compared the two techniques, self-injectors of a combination of papaverine
and phentolamine had a 59 percent dropout rate and a
most frequent side effect of plaquelike nodules in the
penis. VCD users had a 16 percent dropout rate and a
most frequent side effect of blocked ejaculation.

- Which technique results in the hardest erection? Research in monkeys suggests that they are equal.

VACUUM ENTRAPMENT DEVICE

The vacuum entrapment device works on the same principle
as the VCD. The difference is that the vacuum is maintained
throughout intercourse and no use is made of a constricting
ring at the base of the penis. This permits a natural flow of
blood. However, it necessitates the wearing of an individually
fitted silicone sheath over the penis during intercourse.

Some health conditions may justify the choice of a vacuum
entrapment device over a VCD. But one cannot help thinking
that if many men have problems with a VCD, how many more
will have them with a vacuum entrapment device.

RINGS

Constricting rings can be placed at various levels along the shaft of the penis in order to maintain an erection. A ring can change a turgid erection into a rigid one. Referred to as "cockrings" in sex ads, their use can be dangerous, because they have the potential to damage erectile tissue inside the penis. Rings should be used only under a doctor's supervision. Only elastic material should be used, never metal or inelastic material.

CHECKPOINT

- A vacuum device is hard to conceal, but it involves no invasive procedures—no drugs, no needles.
- It works for three out of four men who try it.
- Almost no side effects are involved.

15

Penile Implants and Vascular Surgery

PENILE IMPLANTS

When men are unwilling or unable to use ingestible drugs, intracavernosal self-injection, or a vacuum constriction device—or if the beneficial effects of these have worn off—a penile implant may restore his powers. Dr. Christine Evans gives implants a 90 percent satisfaction rate for men, and an 85 percent rate for their partners. She says that the needs and wishes of a man's spouse are a primary consideration before implantation, since an implant is not worth the trouble if it's not going to be used. In Britain, the choice of implant is usually influenced by cost.

In the United States, penile prosthetic surgery became an accepted procedure in the early 1970s. More than 25,000 penile prostheses were implanted each year in the late 1980s, with a satisfaction rate of about 90 percent. Since the introduction of intracavernosal self-injection, however, the annual number of implantations has declined dramatically.

Having an implant does not interfere with a man's ability to ejaculate and have an orgasm. In fact, in some cases where this ability has been lost, the implant has restored it.

Counseling, both before and after surgery, is regarded as essential to implant success. In counseling before surgery, it is emphasized that an implant usually will not save a deteriorating relationship. Dr. Dudley Seth Danoff emphasizes that, for him, implantation is a treatment of last resort. He notes that if the implants are not long enough, the erect penis will have a floppy tip, like the droopy nose of the Concorde supersonic jet. Dr. Danoff mentions a typical patient that he routinely discourages from having an implant. This patient is an 80-year-old retired man who says he "can't get it up anymore" and wants an implant like the one Dr. Danoff gave his friend. Upon questioning the man, Dr. Danoff discovers that he is in reasonably good health but that his emotional life has been barren for decades. In other words, there is nothing wrong with him that a new zest for life would not cure.

Before agreeing to an implant, a urologist seeks to ensure that the cause of his patient's impotence is physical rather than psychological. Obviously, if the cause is psychological, the urologist would be fixing something that ain't broke. Furthermore, if the psychological problem remains unconfronted, there is a likelihood that a problem will reemerge, regardless of the mechanical success of the implant.

According to Dr. Evans, a man may begin using his implant a month after its insertion, although postoperative discomfort can continue beyond this time. The high level of complaints, however, paints a less pleasant picture. According to 1989 American data, reoperations caused by extrusion or failure of the device occurred in 14 to 44 percent of implants, and infections occurred in 1 to 9 percent of implants. It is reasonable to assume that improvements have been made during the years that have elapsed since then.

Every implant involves the placement of a pair of rods or cylinders in the paired corpora cavernosa of the penis. Present-day penile implants come in two basic types: malleable semirigid rod and inflatable. There are three kinds of inflatable implants, making a total of four choices available.

Malleable Semirigid Rod

This implant consists of a pair of semirigid rods, made of polyethylene, silicone, or a similar material, that can be bent or straightened at will. The two rods are surgically placed in the corpora cavernosa of the penis. Once they are in place, the penis has a permanent erection. The penis can be bent to make it lie close to the body, making it unnoticeable in all but tight swimming trunks or jockey shorts. Straightening the penis with one hand readies it for intercourse in seconds.

The rod is cheaper than the inflatable prosthesis, and, according to Dr. Steven Morganstern, its surgical implantation is simpler and may not involve a hospital stay. With fewer parts, there is less to go wrong with the rod. Another plus is that no pumping is required before intercourse, as with the inflatable, and no deflation after intercourse. On the downside, a permanent erection sooner or later is bound to cause some embarrassing incidents. Additionally, the semirigid rod does not add to either the length or girth of the penis.

Self-Contained Inflatable Implant

This simple kind of inflatable implant has been marketed since 1984 and is composed of, instead of rods, two cylinders filled with fluid. After implantation, there is no permanent erection and the flaccid penis looks natural. Squeezing the cylinder ends nearest the penis tip transfers fluid to a central chamber in each cylinder. Filling the central chamber makes the penis rigid, resulting in an erection similar to that of the semirigid rod. Bending the penis over a finger for ten seconds and then releasing it causes detumescence.

Although more costly than the semirigid rod, the self-contained inflatable implant is cheaper than the two other kinds of inflatable implant. According to Dr. Morganstern, its surgical implantation is comparable to that of the rod. Its obvious advantage over the rod is the absence of a permanent erection. Compared to other inflatable implants, however, the self-contained kind delivers a less rigid erection and there is no increase in penile length or girth. Another drawback is that this kind of implant can occasionally, during intercourse, revert the penis to flaccidity.

Two-Piece Inflatable Implant

In this kind of implant, which has been marketed since 1988, the two penis cylinders are hollow and the fluid is contained in a separate reservoir. This reservoir and a tiny pump are placed in a bulb-shaped chamber, which is surgically located within the scrotum, and connected to the cylinders by two flexible plastic tubes.

Dr. Morganstern says that the two-piece inflatable implant provides a much more natural looking erection than either the self-contained kind or the semirigid rod. But its surgical implantation is more complex, and there are more parts to go wrong.

Three-Piece Inflatable Implant

Dr. Morganstern recommends advanced models of this kind, saying that they offer the best erection of any penile implant and increase both the length and girth of an erection. Two hollow cylinders are placed within the penis, a pump and valves are placed inside the scrotum, and a spherical fluid reservoir is placed in the lower abdomen. All three elements are connected by tubes.

To achieve an erection, a man squeezes the pump inside his scrotum a few times. This causes fluid to be pumped from the reservoir into the two cylinders. An erection results. To cause detumescence, he presses a release valve on the pump and the fluid returns to the reservoir. While this implant has great advantages over the others, it is more costly, requires more complex surgery, and has more parts to malfunction.

VASCULAR SURGERY

Surgical solutions for impotence have been used for only two decades and have nearly all involved the vascular system. Neurological surgery for impotence is still in its infancy. Vascular surgery is of two kinds, venous and arterial.

Vein Surgery

Blood enters the penis by way of arteries, and exits by way of veins. The urological test of cavernosography can help diagnose when impotence is due to leakage of blood from the erectile tissue by way of veins. Once the veins have been located through the contrast of injected fluid on x-ray film, they can be surgically sealed off. Penile vein surgery was first performed to relieve priapism rather than impotence.

Artery Surgery

This is often called revascularization surgery and has been more problematical than vein surgery. The challenge is to provide new channels of blood supply when arteries have become clogged or blocked. The bypass—a penile equivalent of the coronary bypass—has not been very successful. According to Dr. Morganstern, this may be for the following reason: While a bypass provides a new major channel for blood, it does not clear all the tiny arteries through which the blood must pass and where the main problem may exist. Additionally, while a coronary bypass may itself become blocked within ten years, a penile bypass can become blocked within six months.

Dr. Morganstern says that the most successful restoration of potency through artery surgery has involved the repair of arteries damaged through injury in young men.

CHECKPOINT

- When all else fails, there are penile implants.
- When one considers the alternative, implants become a more interesting prospect.
- Recent implant models are very much improved.

16

Other Male
Sexual Dysfunctions

PREMATURE EJACULATION

With this condition, a man ejaculates during foreplay, on first entering, or during the first few thrusts. Premature ejaculation is usually thought of in terms of young men who are novices at sex, are tormented by hormones, and have yet to learn some physical self-control. (The so-called numbing creams that you see in magazine ads as cures for premature ejaculation are usually useless and sometimes dangerous.) But older men can suffer from premature ejaculation, too. Urologists regard it as a disorder that needs treatment when it starts occurring once in every four times a man has sex. But if premature ejaculation suddenly begins to occur in an older man who has never been bothered by it before, he should regard it as a possible symptom of something else and not wait for it to disappear or get worse. Premature ejaculation can have either a physical or psychological cause.

The usual physical cause is prostatitis, which is infection of the prostate gland. Because of the location of the prostate, this is not an easy condition for a doctor to diagnose. The only way he can be sure is by massaging the prostate, with a finger through the rectum, until prostatic fluid emerges from the urethra at the tip of the penis. Lab tests are then performed on the fluid to detect infective agents.

You can possibly avoid that test by looking out for symptoms yourself that a doctor will not have the opportunity to see. Dr. Steven Morganstern lists the following five symptoms for self-diagnosis of prostatis.

- A milky discharge from the urethra at the tip of the penis, not to be confused with semen
- Traces of blood in semen
- A burning sensation in the penis while urinating
- An increase in the number of times you have to urinate during the night
- Unintended stops and starts of the urinary stream, along with a lessening of the urinary flow

These symptoms, he cautions, could mean an infection of the urinary system rather than the prostate.

Antibiotics are used to treat prostatitis. Having sex while under treatment with the antibiotics helps clear the infection, although with some infections sex can be painful. You need to wear a condom to ensure that you are not passing on the infective agent to your partner. To avoid the possibility of a new infection, Dr. Morganstern recommends taking some simple precautions to deter bacteria in feces as a cause. Wash your hands with soap after defecating and wear a condom during anal sex.

When the cause of premature ejaculation is thought to be emotional or psychological, the answer may be Prozac. It is a reflection on the complexity of mood-altering medications that a drug blamed for one sexual problem, as Prozac has been for potency problems, can be recommended as a cure for another sexual problem. Earlier, Masters and Johnson developed a sexual technique to combat the condition.

RETROGRADE EJACULATION

This condition exists when, during orgasm, the semen is not ejaculated but, instead, travels in the opposite direction into the bladder. The condition is caused by failure of the valve that shuts off the urinary passage during sexual activity. The semen in the bladder is later voided from the body with urine, and no threat to health is involved. Because the pleasurable feelings of orgasm remain, the presence of this condition may go undetected for some time.

Having this condition makes it extremely difficult, but not impossible, for a man to have children. Small quantities of sperm can find their way through the urethra and emerge from the tip of the penis, even without an ejaculation. Therefore, retrograde ejaculation cannot be depended on as a natural method of birth control.

The valve in question is a muscle sphincter. It may not be working normally because of damage to the spinal cord or nerves near the bladder. Prostate surgery can also cause the sphincter to malfunction, and, in a small number of cases, so too can the mood-altering drug thioridazine.

Since retrograde ejaculation is not a health-threatening condition, no pharmaceutical or surgical therapies have been developed for it. Men with this condition who wish to have children can have their sperm filtered from their urine to artificially inseminate their spouses. The technique has proved effective.

EJACULATORY FAILURE

Inability to ejaculate, even after prolonged intercourse or masturbation, has no certain cause and no certain cure. It is not a frequent condition. Various theories about its causes have been offered, only to be disproved. A combination of physical and psychological causes remains a possibility. But the condition does not seem to be particularly associated with either circumscision or a puritanical upbringing, as has been believed. Mood-altering drugs, cardiovascular problems, and prostate tumors have also been suggested as causes. Masters and Johnson developed a sexual position to treat this disorder.

PAINFUL EJACULATION

Pain during ejaculation may be a symptom of prostatitis or seminal vesicle infection. The seminal vesicles supply seminal fluid, along with the prostate. If the pain is accompanied by a penile discharge that is not semen, you should see a doctor right away. The doctor will treat an infection with antibiotics. The symptoms to look for in a prostate infection are mentioned in the section on premature ejaculation in this chapter.

Because of the way messages are transported along our nerves and processed inside our brain, the sensation of low levels of pain and pleasure can be confused. An abrupt, powerful sensation can be mistaken for pain. But if you feel strong pain when you ejaculate, you know it. Have it seen to by a doctor. Not having sex because of the pain can lead to emotional potency problems further down the line.

Final Word

The body is naturally healthy and has a homeostasis (balance) that, if allowed to exist, maintains a condition of good health. Lowering our risk factors for impotence in particular, and for overall health in general, edges us closer to that point of balance. We gain huge health returns from certain minimal precautions. By avoiding a few destructive things and keeping persistent ailments under firm management, we can go far toward ensuring ongoing physical and emotional well-being.

A physician can help us overcome an immediate problem. But once that is behind us, it is up to us—not our doctor!—to look out for our health. No matter what therapy we use to combat a potency problem, we need to incorporate that technique into our life in a tranquil, rewarding way, rather than in a furtive, stressful manner. Such advice is easy to give, but harder to follow. There's no denying that it can be a challenge. But a challenge is what it is—not an impossible difficulty that is a further cause of distress.

Forget the studs, gigolos, and Casanovas! The unsung heroes of male sexual life are the quiet men who overcome the challenge of impotence and go on to lead highly pleasurable, sexually powerful lives with a happy and physically satisfied partner.

Where to Get Help

In this new age of competition between large medical centers, free guidance and advice are available as never before. The information is often available by phone. (If the phone call involves a special charge, check the credentials of who you are calling.) Local newspapers and regional magazines frequently carry articles and ads that may be helpful. The Internet teems with information and personal opinion. Men's potency problems have finally emerged as a subject fit for media scrutiny and polite conversation!

The telephone numbers and addresses provided here are by no means a complete listing. The presence or absence of any particular organization on this list should not be taken as an endorsement or lack of one. When writing to an address and expecting a reply, always enclose a stamped, self-addressed envelope.

WALK-IN CLINICS

ICA

ICA stands for Impotence Centers of America, but you won't see it spelled out on any signs or on the door. Discretion and an all-male staff distinguish these walk-in clinics. In mid-1996, they were located only in the New York–New Jersey metropolitan area, but plans were under way to open nationally.

175

Men's Health Centers

These walk-in clinics in mid 1996 were at Boston University Medical Center (where noted urologist Dr. Irwin Goldstein presides) and in the Florida cities of Miami, Boca Raton, Palm Beach Gardens, and Sunrise.

PROFESSIONAL ORGANIZATIONS

American Urological Association
1120 North Charles St., Baltimore, MD 21201
(410) 727-1100

This is the most important professional society of urologists. The association has eight regional sections, and the AUA will direct you to the one closest to you.

American Association of Sex Educators, Counselors and Therapists
P.O. Box 238, Mount Vernon, IA 52314
(319) 895-6407

The AASECT can send you a list of local therapists.

COMPANY-SPONSORED INFORMATION

Pharmacia & Upjohn
(800) 867-7075

P&U can send you a list of local urologists who specialize in male potency problems.

Impotence Information Center
American Medical Systems
Minneapolis, MN 55440
(800) 543-9632

The IIC, part of Pfizer pharmaceutical company, offers general information and local contacts.

Osborn Medical Systems
P.O. Box 1478, Augusta, GA 30903
(800) 438-8592

Osborn supplies general information and details on the vacuum constriction devices that it manufactures.

Palisades Pharmaceutical
64 North Summit St., Tenafly, NJ 07670
(800) 237-9083

Palisades makes yohimbine under the brand name of Yocon and provides information on that drug and where to receive it in treatment.

SUPPORT GROUPS

Impotence Institute of America
2020 Pennsylvania Av., NW, Suite 292, Washington, DC 20006
(800) 669-1603

This nonprofit institute runs Impotence Anonymous, which is loosely organized along the lines of Alcoholics Anonymous and which has scores of local chapters. The institute can tell you how to contact the one nearest you.

Recovery of Male Potency (ROMP)
ROMP Center, Grace Hospital
18700 Meyers Road, Detroit, MI 48235
(800) TEL ROMP; in Michigan, (313) 927-3219

Not for Men Only
Mercy Hospital and Medical Center

Stevenson Expressway at King Drive, Chicago, IL 60616
(312) 567-5567

This support group is linked with the local chapter of Impotence Anonymous.

Potency Restored
Dr. Guilio Scarzella, Montgomery Center, Suite 218
8630 Fenton St., Silver Spring, MD 20910
(301) 588-5777

Urologist Dr. Scarzella runs this local support group for couples.

MEDICAL INFORMATION

American Foundation for Urologic Disease
300 West Pratt St., Suite 401, Baltimore MD 21201-2463
(800) 242-2383

National Kidney and Urologic Diseases Information Clearinghouse
3 Information Way, Bethesda, MD 20892-3580

American Board of Urology
(313) 649-9720

PROSTATE

Prostate Health Council
300 West Pratt St., Baltimore, MD 21201-2463

US TOO
(800) 808-7866

American Prostate Society
(800) 308-1106

NCI
(800) 422-6237

American Cancer Society
1599 Clifton Road, NE, Atlanta, GA 30329
(800) ACS-2345

Prostate Cancer Support Groups Network
300 West Pratt St., Suite 401, Baltimore, MD 21202
(800) 828-7866

SURROGATE SEX PARTNERS

Professional Surrogates Association
(213) 469-4720

The PSA makes contacts internationally.

Stephanie Wadell
Bay Area Surrogate Association
P.O. Box 60971, Palo Alto, CA 94306

She can supply a list of therapists who work with surrogates.

PROSEXUAL DRUG INFORMATION

John Morgenthaler and Dan Joy
(800) LIFE-873

Authors (*Better Sex Through Chemistry*) and editors who are well-known advocates.

MASSAGE THERAPY

American Massage Therapy Association
(708) 864-0123

The AMTA can provide you with the names of local qualified therapists. Currently, nineteen states license massage therapists. With unlicensed therapists, you take your chances.

INTERNET

Impotence Information Page
http://www.demon.co.uk/herniaInfo/mcd.html

These three paperbacks, listed in alphabetical order, will help you find medical information online.

> *Dr. Tom Linden's Guide to Online Medicine* (McGraw-Hill)
>
> *Health Online* by T. Ferguson, M.D. (Addison-Wesley)
>
> *Infomedicine* by F.D. Baldwin and S. McInerney (Little, Brown)

SLEEP APNEA

The American Sleep Apnea Association
2025 Pennsylvania Ave., NW, Suite 905, Washington, DC 20006
(202) 293-3650

National Heart, Lung and Blood Institute Information Center
P.O. Box 30105, Bethesda, MD 20824-0105
(301) 251-1222

Background Reading

American Heart Association Brand Name Fat and Cholesterol Counter, 2d ed., New York: Times Books, 1995.

American Heart Association Cookbook, 5th ed., New York: Ballantine, 1994.

B. Anderson et al., *Getting in Shape: Workout Programs for Men & Women*, Bolinas, Calif.: Shelter, 1994.

F. D. Baldwin and S. McInerney, *Infomedicine: A Consumer's Guide to the Latest in Medical Research*, Boston: Little, Brown, 1996.

L. Bannon, "How a risky surgery became a profit center for some L.A. doctors: Penile enlargements," *Wall Street Journal*, June 6, 1996.

A. H. Bennett, ed., *Impotence: Diagnosis and Management of Erectile Dysfunction*, Philadelphia: Saunders, 1994.

W. I. Bennett et al. (eds.), *Your Good Health: How to Stay Well, and What to Do When You're Not*, Mount Vernon, N.Y.: Consumers Union, 1987.

B. Bilger, "Forever young: Can DHEA temper the ravages of time?" *The Sciences*, pp. 26–30, Sept./Oct. 1995.

D. Bosco, *The People's Guide to Vitamins and Minerals from A to Zinc*, rev. ed., Chicago: Contemporary Books, 1980.

J. E. Brody, "Heart patients need not fear sex, study finds," *New York Times*, May 8, 1996.

———,"Personal health: When depression lifts but sex suffers," *New York Times*, May 15, 1996.

———,"Personal health: When sleep is a nightly struggle to breathe," *New York Times*, May 1, 1996.

N. Bruning, *The Natural Health Guide to Antioxidants*, New York: Bantam, 1994.

L. Caldwell, "Is male menopause myth or reality?" *Men's Fitness*, pp. 102–4, July 1994.

M. Castleman, "A skeptic's guide to aphrodisiacs," *Men's Fitness*, pp. 38–42, August 1995.

J. C. K. Chan et al., "Five- to seven-year follow-up of patients in a pharmacologic erection program: Satisfaction and complications," *J.Urol.*, 147(suppl.):309A, 1992.

M. Chase, "Health journal: New allergy therapies try to halt reactions before they start," *Wall Street Journal*, May 6, 1996.

T. Colborn, D. Dumanoski, and J. P. Myers, *Our Stolen Future*, New York: Dutton, 1996.

L. Cole, "Build a better orgasm," *Men's Fitness*, pp. 53-55, April 1996.

C. Crossen, "Fright by the numbers: Alarming disease data are frequently flawed," *Wall Street Journal*, April 11, 1996.

S. L. Crowley, "Tough love for hearts [Dean Ornish]," *AARP Bulletin*, May 1996.

D. S. Danoff, *Superpotency: How to Get It, Use It, and Maintain It for a Lifetime*, New York: Warner, 1993.

M. Davids, "Doctor's orders: Get a massage," R_x *Remedy*, pp. 30–35, March/April 1996.

DSM-IV: Diagnostic and Statistical Manual of Mental Disorders, 4th ed., Washington, D.C.: American Psychiatric Association, 1995.

M. Ellenberg, "Sexual dysfunction in diabetic patients," *Ann. Intern. Med.*, 92:331, 1980.

S. L. Engel-Arieli, *How Your Body Works*, Emeryville, Calif.: Ziff-Davis Press, 1994.

C. Evans, "Success with erectile dysfunction," *Practitioner*, 239(1554):534–37, 1995.

H. A. Feldman et al., "Impotence and its medical and psychosocial correlates: Results of the Massachusetts Male Aging Study," *J. Urol.*, 151:54–61, 1994.

T. Ferguson, *Health Online: How to Go Online to Find Health Information, Support Forums, and Self-Help Communities in Cyberspace*, Reading, Mass.: Addison-Wesley, 1996.

J. Freid, "It's better when you swallow," *Details*, pp. 74–76, May 1996.

M. L. Gaynor, *Healing Essence: A Cancer Doctor's Practical Program for Hope and Recovery*, New York: Kodansha, 1995.

G. S. Gerber and L. A. Levine, "Pharmacological erection program using prostaglandin E1," *J. Urol.*, 146:786–89, 1991.

S. Gilbert, "Fitness helps, even for smokers," *New York Times*, July 17, 1996.

J. M. Gorman, *The Essential Guide to Psychiatric Drugs*, New York: St. Martin's Press, 1990.

F. E. Govier et al., "Experience with triple-drug therapy in a pharmacological erection program," *J. Urol.*, 150:1822–24, 1993.

A. Gray et al., "Results of the Massachusetts Male Aging Study," *J. Clin. Endocrinol. Metab.*, 71:1442, 1990.

A. C. Guyton, *Basic Neuroscience: Anatomy and Physiology*, Philadelphia: Saunders, 1987.

M. Hirshkowitz et al., "Hypertension, erectile dysfunction, and occult sleep apnea," *Sleep*, 12:223, 1989.

Y. M. Ibrahim, "Village in Finland faces a gold rush fed by margarine," *New York Times*, July 23, 1996.

L. Jaroff, "The man's cancer," *Time*, pp. 58-65, April 1, 1996.

D. Jehl, "Of college girls betrayed and vile chewing gum," *New York Times*, July 10, 1996.

J. Kabat-Zinn, *Wherever You Go, There You Are: Mindfulness Meditation in Everyday Life*, New York: Hyperion, 1994.

A. C. Kinsey et al., *Sexual Behavior in the Human Male*, Philadelphia: Saunders, 1948.

J. Kita, "Substitute teachers," *Men's Health*, pp.107-11, May 1996
———,"Your privates: An owner's manual," *Men's Health*, pp. 90–97, March 1996.

G. Kolata, "Chemicals that mimic hormones spark alarm and debate," *New York Times*, March 19, 1996.

M. Korda, *Man to Man: Surviving Prostate Cancer*, New York: Random House, 1996.

R. J. Krane et al., "Impotence: Medical progress," *N. Engl. J. Med.*, 321:1648–59, 1989.

R. Langreth, "High anxiety: Rivals threaten Prozac's reign," *Wall Street Journal*, May 9, 1996.

T. Linden and M.L. Kienholz, *Dr. Tom Linden's Guide to Online Medicine*, New York: McGraw-Hill, 1995.

O. I. Linet, F. G. Ogrinc et al., "Efficacy and safety of intracavernosal alprostadil in men with erectile dysfunction," *New Engl. J. Med.*, 334(14):873–77, 1996.

L. I. Lipshultz, "Injection therapy for erectile dysfunction," *New Engl. J. Med.*, 334(14):913–14, 1996.

C. Lockie, *Practitioner*, 239:533, 1995.

K. McLeod, "If your doctor prescribes an ACE inhibitor," R_x *Remedy*, pp. 16–21, May/June 1996.

J. B. McKinley and H.A. Feldman, "Results from the Massachusetts Male Aging Study," in A. Rossi (ed.), *Proceedings of the MacArthur Foundation Research Network on Successful Mid-Life Development*, 1992.

W. H. Masters, V.E. Johnson and R.C. Kolodny, *Heterosexuality*, New York: HarperPerennial, 1996.

"A microwave treatment for enlarged prostates," *New York Times*, May 7, 1996.

E. Mindell, *Earl Mindell's Anti-Aging Bible*, New York: Fireside, 1996.

———, *Earl Mindell's Food as Medicine*, New York: Fireside, 1994

D. K. Montague, ed., *Disorders of Male Sexual Function*, Chicago: Year Book Medical Publishers, 1988.

A. Morales et al., "Oral and topical treatment of erectile dysfunction," *Urol. Clin. North Am.*, 22(4):833–45, 1995.

S. Morganstern and A. Abrahams, *Overcoming Impotence: A Doctor's Proven Guide to Regaining Sexual Vitality*, Englewood Cliffs, N.J.: Prentice-Hall, 1994.

J. Morgenthaler and W. Block, "Hunting down the aging clock: An interview with William Regelson, M.D. [on DHEA]," *Life Enhancement News*, October 1995.

M. T. Murray, *The Healing Power of Herbs*, 2d ed., Rocklin, Calif.: Prima, 1995.

"NIH Consensus Development Panel on Impotence, Impotence: NIH Consensus Conference," *JAMA*, 270(1):83–90, 1993.

P. Ody, *The Complete Medicinal Herbal*, New York: Dorling Kindersley, 1993.

D. Ornish, *Dr. Dean Ornish's Program for Reversing Heart Disease*, New York: HarperColllins, 1990.

——, *Eat More, Weigh Less*, New York: HarperCollins, 1993

——, *Everyday Cooking with Dr. Dean Ornish*, New York: HarperCollins, 1996.

R. A. Pascualy and S. W. Soest, *Snoring and Sleep Apnea*, New York: Raven Press, 1994.

S. Perrine, "Secrets of the male orgasm," *Glamour*, pp. 172–75, February 1996.

Physicians' Desk Reference (PDR), 50th ed., Montvale, N.J.: Medical Economics, 1996.

W. Pierpaoli and W. Regelson, *The Melatonin Miracle: Nature's Age-Reversing, Disease-Fighting, Sex-Enhancing Hormone*, New York: Simon & Schuster, 1995.

V. Pitman, *Herbal Medicine*, Rockport, Mass.: Element, 1994.

C. A. Rinzler, "Food for Love: How what you eat affects your libido," *Men's Fitness*, pp. 44–45, May 1994.

M. Roman, "Full stream ahead [prostatitis]," *Men's Health*, pp. 62–64, June 1995

I. Rosenfeld, *Doctor, What Should I Eat? Nutrition Prescriptions for Ailments in Which Diet Can Really Make a Difference*, New York: Random House, 1995.

I. Rosenfeld, *Symptoms*, New York: Simon & Schuster, 1989

R. Santen, ed., *Male Reproductive Dysfunction*, New York: Dekker, 1986.

R. M. Sapolsky, *Why Zebras Don't Get Ulcers: A Guide to Stress, Stress-Related Diseases, and Coping*, New York: Freeman, 1994.

J. Scala, *Prescription for Longevity: Eating Right for a Long Life*, New York: Dutton, 1992.

B. Sears with B. Lawren, *The Zone*, New York: ReganBooks, 1995

J. Sheehan, "Romance prescription," *Longevity*, February 1996.

R. Sikora et al., *Ginkgo biloba* extract in the therapy of erectile dysfunction, *J. Urol.*, 141:188A, 1989.

L. W. Smith, "Defensive sex," *Men's Fitness*, pp. 22–24, September 1993.

A. Smyth, *The Complete Home Healer*, HarperSanFrancisco, 1994

L. Snowdon and M. Humphreys, *Walk Aerobics*, Woodstock, N.Y.: Overlook, 1995.

S. Sobel, "How you choose to live is all that counts," *Advance for Medical Laboratory Professionals*, April 1, 1996.

C. Steele, Helping patients to stop smoking, *The Practitioner*, 239:154–59, 1995.

J. Waynberg, "Aphrodisiacs: Contribution to the clinical validation of the traditional use of *Ptychopetalum guyanna*," *First International Congress on Ethnopharmacology*, Strasbourg, France, June 5–9, 1990.

D. Webster, "Erections 'R' Us," *Men's Health*, pp. 108–13, June 1996

A. Weil, *Health and Healing*, Boston: Houghton Mifflin, 1983; paperback ed., 1995.

R. Winslow, "Pfizer explores treatment for impotence [Viagra]," *Wall Street Journal*, May 6, 1996.

Index